Student Success in Physiology – SBAs and EMQs

HELEN BUTLER
MA (Oxon), MBBS, DRCOG
Academic Foundation Year 2 Trainee
North West London Hospitals NHS Trust
North West Thames Foundation School

Edited by
NEEL SHARMA
BSc (Hons), MBChB, MSc
Core Medical Trainee
Guy's and St Thomas' NHS Foundation Trust,
Honorary Clinical Lecturer
Centre for Medical Education Barts and the
London School of Medicine and Dentistry

Foreword by
TIAGO VILLANUEVA
General Practitioner
Former BMJ Clegg Scholar
Past Editor of the Student BMJ

Radcliffe Publishing
London • New York

Radcliffe Publishing Ltd
33–41 Dallington Street
London
EC1V 0BB
United Kingdom

www.radcliffehealth.com

British Library Cataloguing in Publication Data

A catalogue record for this book is available from the British Library.

ISBN-13: 978 184619 514 3

The paper used for the text pages of this book is FSC® certified. FSC (The Forest Stewardship Council®) is an international network to promote responsible management of the world's forests.

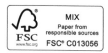

Typeset by Darkriver Design, Auckland, New Zealand
Printed and bound by TJ International Ltd, Padstow, Cornwall, UK

Contents

Foreword

Physiology is one of those extremely important pre-clinical courses that is vital in understanding more advanced fields such as pharmacology and pathophysiology. Mastering it will certainly stand you in good stead during your clinical years and subsequent practice as a doctor. Medical students should thus take sufficient time to learn it well. And I can't think of a better exam preparation port-of-call than Helen Butler and Neel Sharma's latest publication. Building on their experience of writing review books for medical students, they have come up with a new powerful learning tool. Encompassing single best answer and extended matching questions, this book covers all the core areas of physiology. Wherever relevant, questions incorporate key physiology principles applied to actual clinical scenarios, which makes reviewing efforts far more enjoyable and worthwhile – certainly a must have on every medical student's book shelf!

Dr Tiago Villanueva
General Practitioner
Former BMJ Clegg Scholar
Past Editor of the *Student BMJ*
June 2012

Preface

As recent medical graduates, we understand all too well the pressures faced during medical school. Lectures, tutorials, never-ending ward rounds, outpatient clinics, coursework assignments and, of course, let us not forget the gruelling end-of-year exams. Trying to retain and, more importantly, understand all the common (and not-so-common) clinical diseases and basic science truly seems an impossible task.

This self-assessment book is designed to help students tackle questions covering all commonly tested aspects of physiology; questions are included in SBA and EMQ formats with relevant, concise explanations as answers.

We sincerely hope that this book is of use in preparing for your forthcoming examinations, and we wish you every success in your future medical careers.

Helen Butler
Neel Sharma
June 2012

About the author

Helen Butler completed her preclinical training at Oxford University, gaining a degree in medical sciences in 2007. She then graduated from Barts and the London School of Medicine in 2010 with distinctions in clinical science and clinical practice.

Helen is currently working as a foundation year two doctor on the Academic Foundation Programme at the North West London Hospitals NHS Trust. She will continue her training on the General Practice Specialty Training Scheme as part of the London Deanery.

About the editor

Neel Sharma graduated from Manchester University School of Medicine in 2007. He completed his foundation training in North East Thames and subsequently undertook a master's degree in gastroenterology.

Neel has a strong interest in medical education, having authored and edited textbooks at both undergraduate and postgraduate level. He is currently a Core Medical Trainee at Guy's and St Thomas' NHS Foundation Trust, Honorary Clinical Lecturer at the Centre for Medical Education Barts and the London School of Medicine and Dentistry, and has been appointed as Honorary Tutor at the Institute of Medical and Health Sciences Education, The University of Hong Kong.

Education and work are the levers to uplift a people. Work alone will not do it unless inspired by the right ideals and guided by intelligence.

WEB Du Bois, 1868–1963

I dedicate this book to my Nana and Grandad, Pamela and Joseph. Thank you for your love and support, and for all your help to get me to where I am today.

HELEN BUTLER

I would like to dedicate this book to my parents, Ravi and Anita, and my sister Ravnita. Without their continued support and encouragement none of this would have truly been possible.

NEEL SHARMA

Questions

Section 1:
Neuromuscular physiology

Single best answer

1   Concerning the autonomic nervous system, preganglionic neurons secrete which of the following neurotransmitters?

a   Adrenaline

b   Noradrenaline

c   Serotonin (5-HT)

d   Acetylcholine

e   Epinephrine

2   Which of the following is facilitated by parasympathetic stimulation?

a   Vasoconstriction of the blood vessels supplying the abdominal viscera

b   Pupillary dilation

c   Secretion of the apocrine glands in the axillae

d   Increase in heart rate and strength of contraction

e   Contraction of the sphincter muscle of the iris

3 Stimulation of which adrenergic receptor subgroup results in bronchodilation?

a α_1

b α_2

c β_1

d β_2

e δ

4 Which receptors are found between the preganglionic and postganglionic neurons?

a Muscarinic

b Nicotinic

c Adrenergic

d β_1

e β_2

5 Which of the following drugs is an example of an acetylcholinesterase inhibitor?

a Neostigmine

b Noradrenaline

c Atropine

d Pilocarpine

e Nicotine

6 The neuronal myelin sheath allows for a higher transmission velocity and provides nutrition to the neuron. Concerning the following cell types, which is responsible for the formation of the myelin sheath in the central nervous system?

a Oligodendrocyte

b Schwann

c Ependymal

d Astrocyte

e Microglial

7 Concerning the following cell types, which is responsible for the formation of the myelin sheath in the peripheral nervous system?

a Oligodendrocyte

b Schwann

c Ependymal

d Astrocyte

e Microglial

8 Which of the following is NOT permeable to the blood–brain barrier?

a Water

b Carbon dioxide

c Alcohol

d Plasma proteins

e Anaesthetics

9 Which of the following occurs as a side effect of muscarinic receptor blockade?

a   Excess salivation

b   Dry mouth

c   Diarrhoea

d   Urinary incontinence

e   Pupillary constriction

10 The basal ganglia contribute to which of the following?

a   Pain sensation

b   Visual attention

c   Taste sensation

d   Motor control

e   All of the above

11 Which of the following is the major inhibitory neurotransmitter in the central nervous system?

a   Glutamate

b   Gamma-aminobutyric acid (GABA)

c   Aspartate

d   Noradrenaline

e   Acetylcholine

12 Which of the following cranial nerves innervates the parotid salivary gland?

a Hypoglossal

b Glossopharyngeal

c Accessory

d Facial

e Vagus

13 Which neurotransmitter is principally found in the nigrostriatal pathway?

a Glutamate

b Gamma-aminobutyric acid (GABA)

c Dopamine

d Adrenaline

e Noradrenaline

14 Long-term potentiation (LTP) is a mechanism behind which of the following?

a Memory

b Postural stability

c Coordination

d Speech

e Vision

15 Which two sensory modalities travel together in the white-matter tracts of the spinal cord?

a Pain and fine touch

b Pain and proprioception

c Proprioception and temperature

d Vision and hearing

e Temperature and pain

16 The resting membrane potential is principally maintained by which of the following?

a $H^+/K^+ATPase$

b $Na^+/K^+ATPase$

c Calcium influx from the sarcoplasmic reticulum

d Na/glucose cotransporter

e Osmosis

17 An image that appears to be out of focus when in the far distance occurs in which condition?

a Glaucoma

b Bitemporal hemianopia

c Astigmatism

d Farsightedness (hyperopia)

e Nearsightedness (myopia)

18 Which of the following statements regarding the cranial nerves is INCORRECT?

a The inferior oblique muscle is innervated by the oculomotor nerve

b The superior oblique muscle is innervated by the trochlear nerve

c The abducens nerve innervates lateral gaze

d The glossopharyngeal nerve supplies taste to the posterior third of the tongue

e The facial nerve supplies the facial muscles of mastication

19 When the patellar tendon is struck with a tendon hammer, it stretches and results in contraction of the rectus femoris. Which of the following carries afferent signals from the muscle spindle to initiate this reflex?

a Ia nerve

b Ib nerve

c γ-Motor neuron

d α-Motor neuron

e β-Motor neuron

20 Anaerobic respiration creates adenosine triphosphate (ATP) from glycolysis. Which of the following is produced as a by-product?

a Oxygen

b Nitrogen

c Lactic acid

d Creatine phosphate

e Adenosine diphosphate (ADP)

21 Which of the following statements is true with regard to a fast glycolytic skeletal muscle fibre?

a The fibres are red in colour

b They have a small diameter to initiate short-term intense contractions

c The synthesis of ATP is brought about by anaerobic respiration

d They are generally fatigue-resistant

e There is a high myoglobin content

22 Muscles are composed of fast and slow muscle fibres. Which of the following statements regarding fast and slow fibres is correct?

a Fast fibres are red in colour because of large amounts of myoglobin

b Slow fibres are adapted for prolonged muscle contraction

c Fast fibres are smaller for quicker release of energy

d Slow fibres have fewer mitochondria than fast fibres

e Slow fibres metabolise anaerobically

23 During periods of starvation, muscle proteins are broken down to supply the body with an energy source. Which of the following statements regarding this biochemical pathway is correct?

a Muscle breakdown results in the release of glucose directly into the bloodstream

b Muscle breakdown provides the liver with glycogen, from which glucose can be formed

c Muscle breakdown supplies the liver with pyruvate for gluconeogenesis

d The liver converts fatty acids into glucose in response to muscle breakdown during periods of starvation

e Gluconeogenesis is catalysed by glucagon in the liver

24 Which of the following statements regarding the length–tension relationship of skeletal muscle contraction is INCORRECT?

a Increasing initial stretch of the muscle results in increased force of contraction up to an optimum length

b When the initial stretch is small and thus muscle length is short, there is overlap of the actin filaments, which interferes with myosin–actin cross-bridge formation

c At lengths greater than optimum, the actin and myosin filaments are pulled too far apart, which results in reduced overlap and thus reduced contraction

d Muscle fibre tension is sensed by Golgi tendon organs and muscle spindles

e The length–tension relationship of contraction is linear, in that the greater the stretch, the greater the tension and the greater the force of muscle contraction

25 Which of the following muscle types has the slowest speed of contraction?

a Cardiac

b Smooth

c Skeletal

d Myosin

e Actin

26 The force of muscle contraction can be increased by 'summation' where a second action potential fires before the muscle fibre has relaxed from the first. A state of quick-fire sequence of action potentials can result in which of the following?

a Paraesthesia

b Wasting

c Clonus

d Paralysis

e Tetany

Extended matching questions

Theme: Physiology of skeletal, cardiac and smooth muscle

a Cardiac muscle

b Smooth muscle

c Skeletal muscle

d Fast fibres

e Slow fibres

f Actin

g Myosin

h Noradrenaline

i Acetylcholine

j Dopamine

k Serotonin

For each of the following questions, select the most appropriate answer from the list of options above. Each option may be used once, more than once or not at all.

1 Which fibres look red in appearance due to their high levels of myoglobin?

2 Which neurotransmitter acts at the neuromuscular junction of skeletal muscle?

3 Which muscle type acts by slow cycling of actin–myosin cross-bridges?

4 Name the thick filament involved in cross-bridge formation of muscle contraction

5 Infarction of this muscle type results in characteristic changes on the electrocardiogram (ECG)

Theme: Neurotransmitters

a   Acetylcholine

b   Dopamine

c   Glutamine

d   Gamma-aminobutyric acid (GABA)

e   Nicotinic receptor

f   Muscarinic receptor

g   α-Receptor

h   β-Receptor

For each of the following questions, select the most appropriate answer from the list of options above. Each option may be used once, more than once or not at all.

1   Name the neurotransmitter at the neuromuscular junction

2   Name a common inhibitory neurotransmitter

3   Which receptor is found at the presynaptic neuron in the sympathetic nervous system?

4   Which receptor is found at the presynaptic neuron in the parasympathetic nervous system?

5   L-Dopa can be given to increase levels of which neurotransmitter?

Theme: The musculoskeletal system

a   Agonist

b   Antagonist

c   Ligament

d   Tendon

e   Smooth muscle

f   Skeletal muscle

g   Cardiac muscle

h   Enthesitis

i   Epicondylitis

j   Myosin

k   Actin

For each of the following questions, select the most appropriate answer from the list of options above. Each option may be used once, more than once or not at all.

1   What is the name of the thick filament of muscle fibres?

2   Which muscle type is comprised of organised rows of fibres with a striated appearance?

3   What is the name of the structure connecting muscle to bone?

4   What is the action of the triceps muscle with regard to elbow flexion?

5   What is the name given to inflammation at the site of tendon or ligament insertion?

Theme: Neuronal transmission

a Relative refractory period

b Absolute refractory period

c Resting membrane potential

d Action potential

e Hyperpolarisation

f Depolarisation

g Repolarisation

For each of the following questions, select the most appropriate answer from the list of options above. Each option may be used once, more than once or not at all.

1 The interval during which repolarisation is occurring, sodium channels are closed and potassium channels open

2 Equivalent to −70 mV with ion gradients maintained by Na^+/K^+ ATPase

3 A rapid impulse occurring once a threshold is reached, resulting in the opening of voltage-activated Na^+ channels

4 The period in which Na^+ channels recover from inactivation, but at which there are an insignificant number of open channels to initiate an action potential

5 The voltage difference between the extracellular and intracellular sides of the cell membrane, at which the intracellular component is negative with respect to the extracellular

Section 2: Cardiovascular and respiratory physiology

Single best answer

1 What is the action of noradrenaline on a vascular α_1-receptor?

   a Vasodilatation

   b Vasoconstriction

   c Decreased vascular resistance

   d Bronchoconstriction

   e Increased vascular permeability

2 Cardiac output is the product of which of the following parameters?

   a Heart rate and total peripheral resistance

   b Systolic and diastolic blood pressure

   c Respiratory rate and preload

   d Afterload and contractility

   e Heart rate and stroke volume

3   The Frank–Starling law states that the force of contraction of the heart is related to which of the following?

a   Heart rate

b   End-diastolic volume

c   Refractory period

d   Respiratory rate

e   Afterload

4   Which of the following is true with regard to the cardiovascular system and altitude?

a   Blood pressure will always increase after acclimatisation to altitude

b   Atmospheric partial pressure of oxygen (pO_2) is higher with increasing altitude, which results in a reduction in respiratory rate

c   Atmospheric partial pressure of carbon dioxide (pCO_2) is lower at increasing altitude, and thus always results in respiratory alkalosis

d   There is an increase in erythropoietin secretion augmenting an increase in red cell production, thus increasing vascular oxygen-carrying capacity

e   The activity of renin increases to stimulate heart rate, which compensates for the lower environmental pO_2

5 Right bundle-branch block, left axis deviation and first-degree heart block on an electrocardiogram (ECG) indicate which of the following?

  a Complete heart block

  b Trifascicular block

  c Diabetes mellitus

  d ECG leads placed in reverse

  e ST-elevation myocardial infarction

6 In a normal healthy heart, where is the origin of electrical activity which regulates the heart rate?

  a Sinoatrial node

  b Atrioventricular node

  c Bundle of His

  d Right ventricle

  e Left ventricle

7 Which of the following correctly describes complete heart block?

  a The sinoatrial node fires at a quicker rate than the atrioventricular node

  b The right ventricle fibrillates independently of the sinoatrial node

  c The heart is in a state of cardiac arrest and defibrillation is required

  d It is a form of pulseless electrical activity (PEA)

  e There is no relationship between atrial and ventricular activity

8 Atrial fibrillation occurs when the atria contract at an irregular rate, a rate which is not governed by the intrinsic pacemaker of the heart. Which of the following occurs more frequently in atrial fibrillation?

   a Scleroderma

   b Systemic lupus erythematosus (SLE)

   c Sick sinus syndrome

   d Sclerosing cholangitis

   e Stroke

9 The T wave on the electrocardiogram (ECG) corresponds to which of the following?

   a Electrical activity leaving the sinoatrial node (SAN)

   b Atrial depolarisation

   c Ventricular repolarisation

   d Atrial repolarisation

   e Electrical activity at the atrioventricular node (AVN)

10 The rate of depolarisation of the sinoatrial node (SAN) can be increased by which of the following?

   a Parasympathetic activity

   b Sympathetic activity

   c Vagal nerve activity

   d β-Blocker (e.g. propranolol) activity

   e Ca-channel blocker (e.g. verapamil) therapy

11 Which of the following most commonly coexists with aortic stenosis?

   a Wide pulse pressure

   b Left ventricular hypertrophy

   c Collapsing pulse

   d Right ventricular dilatation

   e Complete heart block

12 Which of the following is true with regard to the ejection fraction of the heart?

   a In a normally functioning heart, one would expect an approximate 33% ejection fraction

   b The ejection fraction describes the remaining volume in the ventricle at the end of systole

   c The ejection fraction is 100% in a normal heart

   d The ejection fraction describes the volume of blood in the ventricle at the end of diastole

   e The ejection fraction can be calculated by dividing the stroke volume by the end-diastolic volume

13 Which of the following increases the risk of atherosclerosis?

   a High cardiac output

   b High protein diet

   c Previous deep vein thrombosis

   d Previous pulmonary embolism

   e Hyperlipidaemia

14 Which of the following is true with regard to the cardiovascular system on standing up?

   a Preload (venous return) to the right atrium increases

   b The parasympathetic nervous system is stimulated, due to the reduction in cardiac output

   c As a result of the reduction in cardiac output and stimulation of a branch of the autonomic nervous system, heart rate increases

   d Peripheral vascular resistance decreases to divert blood away from the peripheries

   e The increase in preload results in an increased stroke volume and cardiac output (as per the Frank–Starling law)

15 Hypoventilation results in which of the following conditions?

   a A reduction in serum bicarbonate

   b Respiratory acidosis

   c Respiratory alkalosis

   d Low arterial CO_2

   e Metabolic alkalosis

16 Concerning lung volumes, which of the following is the correct definition of 'residual volume'?

   a The volume of gas in the lungs after a normal expiration

   b The volume of gas in the lungs after a maximal expiration

   c The amount of gas inhaled or exhaled during a normal breath

   d The volume of the lungs at the end of a maximal inspiratory effort

   e The amount of gas that can be inhaled by a maximal inspiratory effort following maximal expiration

17 Whose law describes airway resistance by the following equation?

Resistance = $\dfrac{8\,\eta l}{\pi r^4}$ (η = viscosity of gas, l = length, r = radius)

a Newton's

b Boyle's

c Ohm's

d Poiseuille's

e None of the above

18 Which of the following statements regarding perfusion of the lungs is correct?

a Oxygenated blood is carried in the pulmonary arteries

b Bronchial veins carry oxygen to supply the lung tissue

c Low oxygen levels cause vasoconstriction of the pulmonary vasculature

d The pulmonary veins receive deoxygenated blood from the vena cavae

e Pulmonary arteries carry oxygenated blood to the lungs

19 Which of the following structures produces surfactant?

a γ-Type I cells

b γ-Type II cells

c α-1-Antitrypsin

d Type I pneumocytes

e Type II pneumocytes

20 Which of the following is true with regard to the function of surfactant?

    a It is a protease inhibitor which prevents alveolar breakdown in smoking-induced emphysema

    b It lines the large airways to facilitate ciliary movement

    c It increases compliance of the lungs by reducing alveolar surface tension

    d It catalyses the conversion of angiotensin I to angiotensin II, which acts to increase fluid and sodium reabsorption in the kidney

    e All of the above

21 Which of the following is true with regard to the effect of smoking on lung function?

    a Smoking is the main risk factor for chronic obstructive pulmonary disease (COPD)

    b Smoking promotes paralysis of cilia and an increased rate of infection

    c There is an increased risk of all types of lung cancers over non-smokers

    d Smoking increases bronchial hyperactivity

    e All of the above

22 Which of the following can be used in the treatment of an acute asthma attack and works by bronchodilation?

    a H_2 antagonist

    b Histamine

    c β_2-Blocker

    d β_1-Agonist

    e β_2-Agonist

23 The oxygen-carrying capacity of haemoglobin can be depicted using the haemoglobin–oxygen dissociation curve, showing the percentage saturation at increasing levels of oxygen partial pressure. What effect does an increased carbon dioxide concentration have on the haemoglobin–oxygen dissociation curve?

a Shift to the right

b Shift to the left

c Shift upward

d Shift downward

e It has no effect

24 In order for carbon dioxide to be carried by erythrocytes, the following reaction occurs:

$$CO_2 + H_2O \leftrightarrow H_2CO_3 \leftrightarrow H^+ + HCO_3^-$$

Which of the following enzymes catalyses this reaction?

a Renin

b Protein kinase C

c Carbonic anhydrase

d Cytochrome P450

e Orotidine 5-phosphate decarboxylase

25 Which of the following changes is detected by central chemoreceptors and results in an increased respiratory rate?

a Increase in pH of cerebrospinal fluid (CSF)

b Decrease in pH of capillary blood

c Decrease in pH of the brain extracellular fluid

d Decrease in arterial pO_2

e Increase in arterial pO_2

26 Which of the following conditions would cause an increase in respiratory rate?

a A rise in temperature

b Opiate toxicity

c A decrease in temperature

d An increase in serum pH

e All of the above

Extended matching questions

Theme: Cardiovascular pharmacology

a Digoxin

b Noradrenaline

c Ca^{2+} channel agonist

d β-Blocker

e Nitric oxide

f Diuretics

g β-Agonist

h Ca^{2+} channel blocker

For each of the following questions, select the most appropriate answer from the list of options above. Each option may be used once, more than once or not at all.

1 Which of a–h acts on the Na^+/K^+ ATPase and can be used in cardiac arrhythmias?

2 Which inotrope acts on both α- and β-adrenergic receptors?

3 Which inotrope derives from the foxglove plant *Digitalis lanata*?

4 Which pharmacological agent is a mildly positive inotrope and a negative chronotrope?

5 Which pharmacological agent is a vasoconstrictor and acts on the β_1 receptor?

Theme: Physiology and structure of the heart

a Right atrium

b Right ventricle

c Left atrium

d Left ventricle

e Sinoatrial node

f Atrioventricular node

g Bundle of His

h Aorta

i Vena cava

For each of the following, select the most appropriate answer from the list of options above. Each option may be used once, more than once or not at all.

1 This vessel carries blood with the highest carbon dioxide concentration (pCO_2)

2 Electrical activity originating here controls the rate of cardiac contraction

3 Fibres in this area transmit depolarisation across the interventricular septum

4 This structure allows the electrical impulse to pass between the atria and ventricles

5 This area has the highest rate of spontaneous electrical activity

Theme: Reversible causes of cardiac arrest

a   Tension pneumothorax

b   Toxins

c   Thromboembolism

d   Tamponade

e   Hypoxia

f   Hypovolaemia

g   Hyperkalaemia

h   Hypothermia

For each of the following scenarios, select the most appropriate cause of cardiac arrest from the list of options above. Each option may be used once, more than once or not at all.

1   A 78-year-old gentleman with extensive gastrointestinal bleeding

2   A 23-year-old lady is in respiratory distress; she has reduced breath sounds on the right side and her trachea is shifted to the left

3   An elderly gentleman is on spironolactone, ramipril and non-steroidal anti-inflammatory drugs (NSAIDs)

4   An 18-year-old girl is found collapsed in a nightclub; she feels warm to touch and has grossly dilated pupils

5   An 80-year-old lady with a history of ischaemic heart disease arrested following complaints of severe, tight chest pain

Theme: Respiratory physiology

a Dead space

b Tidal volume

c Increase

d Decrease

e Aortic bodies

f Carotid bodies

g Respiratory acidosis

h Respiratory alkalosis

i Metabolic alkalosis

For each of the following questions, select the most appropriate answer from the list of options above. Each option may be used once, more than once or not at all.

1 Equivalent to approximately 500 mL, the volume of air which moves into and out of the lungs during normal breathing at rest

2 Equivalent to approximately 150 mL, the volume of air inspired which does not play a role in gaseous exchange

3 Hyperventilation results in which acid–base condition?

4 What is the effect of acidosis on respiratory rate?

5 What is the effect of alkalosis on respiratory rate?

Section 3: Gastrointestinal and metabolism

Single best answer

1 Which of the following is NOT a gastrointestinal hormone?

   a Cholecystokinin

   b Secretin

   c Gastric inhibitory peptide

   d Gastrin

   e Atrial natriuretic peptide

2 Which of the following is required for the absorption of vitamin B_{12}?

   a Vitamin B_1

   b Vitamin C

   c Intrinsic factor

   d Factor V Leiden

   e Parietal factor

3   Which of the following pathways correctly outlines the detoxification of alcohol by the liver?

a   Ethanol → acetaldehyde → acetate

b   Ethanol → acetyldehydrogenase

c   Methanol → acetate

d   Ethanol → acetazolamide

e   Methanol → acetyldehydrogenase → methane

4   Synthetic function of the liver is best assessed looking at which of the following parameters?

a   Haemoglobin

b   Albumin

c   Gamma-glutamyl transpeptidase (γGT)

d   Alanine transaminase (ALT)

e   Aspartate transaminase (AST)

5   Chief cells of the stomach are responsible for the secretion of which of the following?

a   Hydrochloric acid

b   *Helicobacter pylori*

c   Pepsinogen

d   Amylase

e   Lipase

6 Which of the following hormones regulates the release of bile from the gall bladder?

   a Cholecystokinin

   b Amylase

   c Lipase

   d Growth hormone

   e Glucagon

7 Hepatic synthesis of which of the following clotting factors is vitamin K–dependent?

   a Prothrombin

   b Factor VII

   c Factor IX

   d Factor X

   e All of the above

8 Post-operatively, patients may experience paralysis of the bowel (ileus). Which of the following electrolyte abnormalities most commonly predisposes to ileus?

   a Hypernatraemia

   b Hyperkalaemia

   c Hyperphosphataemia

   d Hypokalaemia

   e Hyperalbuminaemia

9 A short length of small bowel (<100 cm), following resection after mesenteric infarction for example, is incapable of absorbing the body's nutritional requirement. Which of the following is most suitable to help meet the nutritional requirements of the body in such a case?

a Nasogastric (NG) feeding

b Nasojejunal (NJ) feeding

c Percutaneous endoscopic gastrostomy (PEG) feeding

d Total parenteral nutrition (TPN)

e All of the above

10 The four cardinal signs of intestinal obstruction include all but which of the following?

a Absolute constipation

b Abdominal pain

c Abdominal distension

d Nausea and vomiting

e Diarrhoea

11 Which transporter results in the secretion of gastric acid into the stomach lumen?

a Na^+/HCO_3^- pump on the luminal membrane of the parietal cell

b H^+/K^+ ATPase on the parietal cell luminal membrane

c Chief cell $Na^+/K^+/Cl^-$ ATPase

d H^+ ATPase

e Chief cell pepsinogen

12 Which of the following is responsible for the secretion of insulin in response to hyperglycaemia?

a α-Cells

b β-Cells

c δ-Cells

d Parietal cells

e Chief cells

13 Which of the following mechanisms promotes gastric secretion?

a Intestinal protein digestion

b Distension of the stomach

c Thought, smell and taste of food

d Options a and b

e Options a, b and c

14 Which of the following can damage gastric mucosa?

a *Helicobacter pylori*

b Non-steroidal anti-inflammatory drugs (NSAIDs)

c Aspirin

d Alcohol

e All of the above

15 Refeeding syndrome can develop with the reintroduction of nutrition after a period of starvation. This condition can be fatal due to a drop in which of the following?

a Potassium

b Phosphate

c Zinc

d Albumin

e Sodium

16 Omeprazole is a proton-pump inhibitor used to reduce gastric acid secretion in gastro-oesophageal reflux and peptic ulcer disease. By which mechanism does the proton-pump inhibitor act?

a Na^+/K^+ ATPase inhibitor

b H^+/K^+ ATPase inhibitor

c Kreb's cycle inhibitor

d G-cell receptor antagonist

e $Na^+/K^+/2Cl^-$ inhibitor

17 Which of the following is correct with regard to splenic function?

a The spleen provides a store of blood

b It acts as a reservoir of erythrocytes

c It has an immunological function and produces lymphocytes in the neonatal period

d The spleen has a phagocytic role in the defence against infection

e All of the above

18 Which of the following mechanisms may lead to malabsorption?

a Overeating and obesity

b Anorexia

c Bulimia

d Chronic alcoholism

e Pregnancy

19 Which of the following drugs would slow bowel motility and thus reduce the output of a small-bowel stoma?

   a Ibuprofen

   b Codeine phosphate

   c Metoclopramide

   d Cyclizine

   e Paracetamol

20 Which of the following parameters will be high in a state of iron deficiency?

   a Iron

   b Ferritin

   c Folate

   d Mean corpuscular volume (MCV)

   e Total iron-binding capacity (TIBC)

21 Which of the following is a monosaccharide commonly found in the diet?

   a Sucrose

   b Starch

   c Glucose

   d Lactose

   e Glycogen

22 Which of the following is true with regard to the production and function of bile salts?

    a Bile salts are produced in the gall bladder

    b Bile salts function to emulsify fats to aid in digestion

    c Bile salts function to digest fats to form fatty acids and glucagon

    d Bile salts are produced in the pancreas

    e Bile salts aid in the digestion of carbohydrates to form micelles

23 Which nerve supplies the muscles of mastication which initiate chewing and the initial breakdown of food?

    a C2

    b Facial

    c Glossopharyngeal

    d Trigeminal

    e Recurrent laryngeal

24 Which of the following is NOT a fat-soluble vitamin?

    a Vitamin E

    b Vitamin K

    c Vitamin D

    d Vitamin C

    e Vitamin A

25 Gastrin is secreted by which cells in the stomach?

a Islets of Langerhans

b Apocrine cells

c Parietal cells

d Chief cells

e G cells

26 Which of the following is true with respect to the sympathetic system and the enterogastric reflex?

a The sympathetic system results in tightening of the pylorus, which prevents gastric content from entering the small intestine

b It acts to increase gastric acid secretion

c The reflex stimulates vagal activity

d It results in relaxation of the pyloric sphincter

e It results in receptive relaxation of gastric smooth muscle

Extended matching questions

Theme: Causes of malabsorption

    a Pancreatic insufficiency

    b Short bowel syndrome

    c Jejunal mucosa atrophy

    d Irradiation mucosal damage

    e Bacterial overgrowth

    f Autoimmunity

    g Extrinsic compression

    h Intraluminal compression

    i Dysmotility

For each of the following conditions, select the most likely cause of malabsorption from the list of options above. Each option may be used once, more than once or not at all.

1 Pernicious anaemia (vitamin B_{12} deficiency)

2 Post-treatment for cervical carcinoma

3 Cystic fibrosis

4 Coeliac disease

5 Post-mesenteric infarct

Theme: Minerals and vitamins

a   Zinc

b   Selenium

c   Phosphate

d   Magnesium

e   Calcium

f   Vitamin B_1

g   Vitamin B_6

h   Vitamin C

i   Vitamin D

j   Vitamin E

For each of the following questions, select the most appropriate answer from the list of options above. Each option may be used once, more than once or not at all.

1   Name a fat-soluble vitamin

2   Deficiency of this water-soluble vitamin can lead to scurvy

3   Its absorption is stimulated by parathyroid hormone (PTH)

4   The commonly used name for thiamine

5   Its metabolism involves the liver, the kidney and the sun

Theme: Functions of the liver

a Ferritin

b Albumin

c Clotting factors

d Transferrin

e Haemoglobin

f Ammonia

g Haemochromatosis

h Hepatitis

i Portal hypertension

For each of the following questions, select the most appropriate answer from the list of options above. Each option may be used once, more than once or not at all.

1 A condition in which there is iron overload, leading to hepatic disease

2 This can result in the formation of varices and life-threatening upper gastrointestinal haemorrhage

3 A reduction in this protein results in oedema and ascites

4 An acute-phase response marker

5 A toxic substance converted into urea by the liver and excreted by the kidneys

Theme: The metabolism of glucose

a   Glycogenolysis

b   Glycogenesis

c   Glycogen

d   Glucose

e   Glucagon

f   Glycerine

g   Glucose 6-phosphate

h   Gluconeogenesis

i   Glycolytic

For each of the following questions, select the most appropriate answer from the list of options above. Each option may be used once, more than once or not at all.

1   The process by which glucose is synthesised from non-carbohydrate substrate

2   The process by which glycogen is broken down into glucose 1-phosphate molecules

3   The process by which glycogen is synthesised for glucose storage

4   The process from which pyruvate is formed from glucose to enter the tricarboxylic acid (or Kreb's) cycle

5   A pancreatic enzyme which catalyses the formation of glucose from glycogen stores

Section 4: Endocrinology and reproduction

Single best answer

1 At which point in the female reproductive cycle does the luteinising hormone (LH) surge occur?

   a Mid-luteal phase

   b Mid-follicular phase

   c 24 hours before ovulation

   d 48 hours after ovulation

   e 7 days before menstruation

2 During the follicular phase, which structure secretes oestrogen?

   a Hypothalamus

   b Posterior pituitary gland

   c Anterior pituitary gland

   d Follicular theca interna cells

   e Corpus luteum

3 Which of the following markers would you expect to be raised in ovarian failure?

a Oestradiol

b Oestriol

c Beta-human chorionic gonadotrophin (β-hCG)

d Progesterone

e Follicle-stimulating hormone (FSH)

4 Which posterior pituitary hormone plays an important role in breast-feeding mothers?

a Follicle-stimulating hormone (FSH)

b Progesterone

c Prolactin

d Oestrogen

e Oxytocin

5 Which of the following is responsible for the production of androgens from cholesterol?

a Sertoli cells

b Leydig cells

c Primordial germ cells

d Seminal vesicles

e Epididymis

6 The pre-emptive administration of steroids to the mother at risk of preterm labour helps in the production of which of the following in the foetus?

   a Immunoglobulins

   b Osteoblasts

   c Myoglobin

   d Amino acids

   e Surfactant

7 Which of the following is true with regard to the menarche?

   a The average age of menarche in the UK is 9 years

   b Thelarche is the point at which breast development occurs

   c The climacteric is the point at which a girl starts to menstruate

   d Delayed puberty is diagnosed if menstruation has not occurred by 15 years of age

   e Secondary amenorrhoea occurs when menstruation ceases for a period of over 6 months in a woman who has menstruated in the past

8 Which of the following electrolyte abnormalities most commonly accompanies primary hypoadrenalism (Addison's disease)?

   a Hypokalaemia

   b Hyponatraemia

   c Hypocalcaemia

   d Hypophosphataemia

   e Hypernatraemia

9 Which of the following controls testosterone production by the Leydig cells?

a Follicle-stimulating hormone (FSH)

b Luteinising hormone (LH)

c Gonadotrophin-releasing hormone (GnRH)

d Endorphin

e Testosterone

10 Which of the following is cleaved from pre-proopiomelanocortin (pre-POMC)?

a Adrenocorticotrophin hormone (ACTH)

b Growth hormone (GH)

c Testosterone

d Thyroid-stimulating hormone (TSH)

e Follicle-stimulating hormone (FSH)

11 Some antipsychotic medications, e.g. chlorpromazine, cause anti-dopaminergic effects. In relation to the hypothalamic–pituitary axis, which of the following is a potential adverse effect of chlorpromazine and the typical antipsychotics?

a Chorea

b Peripheral neuropathy

c Diarrhoea

d Palpitations

e Gynaecomastia

12 Which of the following can be detected in the urine to confirm pregnancy?

a Leucocytes

b Beta-human chorionic gonadotrophin (β-hCG)

c Glucose

d Protein

e Luteinising hormone (LH)

13 Which of the following can be detected in the urine to predict ovulation?

a Leucocytes

b Beta-human chorionic gonadotrophin (β-hCG)

c Glucose

d Protein

e Luteinising hormone (LH)

14 Unopposed oestrogen therapy (i.e. oestrogen administration without progesterone) increases the risk of which of the following?

a Ectopic pregnancy

b Polycystic ovarian syndrome

c Osteoporosis

d Transitional cell carcinoma

e Endometrial carcinoma

15 Hormone replacement therapy (HRT) reduces the incidence of which of the following?

a Ectopic pregnancy

b Polycystic ovarian syndrome

c Osteoporosis

d Transitional cell carcinoma

e Endometrial carcinoma

16 What name is given to the last 14 days of the menstrual cycle?

a Proliferative phase

b Secretory phase

c Ovulatory phase

d Implantation

e Menstruation

17 Hormones that travel via the extracellular fluid to act on local cells are known as which of the following?

a Paracrine

b Autocrine

c Endocrine

d Allocrine

e Neuroendocrine

18 Pituitary hypersecretion of growth hormone (GH) in the adult leads to which of the following conditions?

a Pituitary dwarfism

b Haemochromatosis

c Acromegaly

d Addison's disease

e Progeria

19 What is the full name of the thyroid hormone T_3?

a Thyroxine

b Thyroid-stimulating hormone (TSH)

c Triiodothyronine

d Iodine

e Triiodothyroxine

20 A prolactinoma results in excess levels of prolactin and menstrual disturbances in women. Where is the most likely origin of the tumour?

a Pituitary

b Thyroid

c Hypothalamus

d Adrenal cortex

e Adrenal medulla

21 Which substance does the parafollicular cells of the thyroid gland secrete?

a Vitamin D

b Triiodothyroxine

c Calcitonin

d Parathyroid hormone

e Aldosterone

22 Which of the following is true with regard to the action of parathyroid hormone (PTH)?

a Triggered by a rise in calcium, PTH increases serum calcium by promoting reabsorption of calcium into the intestine and bone

b PTH results in the release of thyroxine to increase basal metabolic rate

c PTH inhibits bone osteoclastic activity, thus increasing serum calcium

d PTH acts to increase blood calcium levels by actions on the renal tubule, intestinal absorption and bone

e PTH inhibits synthesis and activation of vitamin D $(1,25\text{-}(OH)_2D_3)$

23 Which of the following is required for the metabolism of vitamin D?

a Infrared waves

b Ultraviolet light

c Vitamin C

d Vitamin K

e Fibre

24 Which cells of the pancreas are responsible for the secretion of glucagon?

a α

b β

c γ

d Acinar

e All of the above

25 Which of the following statements is true with regard to the thyroid axis?

a Thyroid-stimulating hormone (TSH) increases thyrotrophin-releasing hormone (TRH) secretion by positive feedback

b TSH decreases TRH production by negative feedback

c TRH decreases TSH and thus thyroxine (T_4) and triiodothyronine (T_3)

d All of the above

e None of the above

26 Which of the following adrenal structures is responsible for the production of mineralocorticoids?

a Adrenal medulla

b Adrenal cortex: zona glomerulosa

c Adrenal cortex: zona fasciculata

d Adrenal cortex: zona reticularis

e Adrenal capsule

Extended matching questions

Theme: The hypothalamic–pituitary axis

a Leptin

b Antidiuretic hormone (ADH)

c Prolactin

d Dopamine

e Gonadotrophin-releasing hormone (GnRH)

f Thyroxine

g Progesterone

h Adrenocorticotrophin hormone (ACTH)

i Growth hormone

For each of the following questions, select the most appropriate answer from the list of options above. Each option may be used once, more than once or not at all.

1 Name a hormone which is produced in the posterior pituitary gland

2 Which hormone tonically inhibits prolactin?

3 Overproduction of this hormone results in hyponatraemia and may occur secondary to small-cell lung cancer

4 Inability to secrete sufficient amounts of this hormone results in cranial diabetes insipidus

5 Which of the above results in the secretion of two hormones from the anterior pituitary gland and is important in the control of the menstrual cycle and fertility?

Theme: The menstrual cycle

a Follicle-stimulating hormone (FSH)

b Luteinising hormone (LH)

c Oestriol

d Progesterone

e Gonadotrophin-releasing hormone (GnRH)

f Oestradiol

g Day 1

h Day 14

i Day 21

j Day 28

k Endometrium

l Ovary

m Myometrium

For each of the following questions, select the most appropriate answer from the list of options above. Each option may be used once, more than once or not at all.

1 Unopposed oestrogen causes hyperplasia of this tissue

2 The final day of an average menstrual cycle

3 Progesterone levels can be measured to confirm ovulation on which day?

4 Which hormone is produced in the hypothalamus?

5 Which hormone is known as the 'pro-pregnancy' hormone?

Theme: Water and electrolyte balance

a   Antidiuretic hormone (ADH)

b   Atrial natriuretic peptide (ANP)

c   Osmolarity

d   Plasma volume

e   Sodium

f   Potassium

g   Furosemide

h   Spironolactone

i   Aldosterone

j   Nitric oxide

For each of the following questions, select the most appropriate answer from the list of options above. Each option may be used once, more than once or not at all.

1   A 1% change in this parameter leads to ADH secretion

2   Name an aldosterone antagonist

3   Name an aldosterone stimulator

4   Name an example of a loop diuretic

5   Which diuretic can lead to hyperkalaemia?

Theme: Diabetes mellitus

a Insulin resistance

b Obesity

c Hypoglycaemia

d Diabetic ketoacidosis

e Type I diabetes mellitus

f Type II diabetes mellitus

g Non-ketotic hyperglycaemia

h Insulin

i Glucagon

j Glycogen

For each of the following questions, select the most appropriate answer from the list of options above. Each option may be used once, more than once or not at all.

1 A complication of type I diabetes mellitus, characterised by ketonuria and extreme hyperglycaemia, which can lead to a depressed conscious level and coma

2 A chronic condition characterised by destruction of β-islet cells and impaired insulin secretion

3 A chronic condition which commonly presents with end-organ complications of the disease, such as retinopathy or peripheral neuropathy

4 Which hormone involved with glycaemic control is secreted by α-cells of the pancreas?

5 Which hormone acts to lower elevated blood glucose, increases protein synthesis and controls glucose and amino acid transport into many cells?

Section 5: Fluid regulation and the kidneys

Single best answer

1 Which of the following is a function of the kidney?

  a Acid–base balance

  b Stimulation of erythropoiesis

  c Regulation of osmolarity

  d Regulation of fluid balance

  e All of the above

2 Which of the following describes the method of epithelial transport at the renal tubule?

  a Ussing's model

  b Bohr's model

  c Hardy's model

  d Walling's model

  e None of the above

3 Which of the following is true with regard to the action of antidiuretic hormone (ADH)?

   a It causes increased sodium secretion at the collecting duct

   b It promotes insertion of aquaporin I vesicles at the collecting duct

   c It reduces the permeability of the inner medullary collecting duct

   d It promotes osmotic diuresis

   e It works at vasopressin (V_2) receptors to generate cAMP and activates protein kinase A (PKA)

4 Which of the following does NOT play a role in the monitoring/detection of the effective circulating volume?

   a Baroreceptors in the aortic arch

   b Stretch receptors in the renal afferent arteriole

   c Macula densa

   d Baroreceptors in the carotid body

   e Osmoreceptors in the hypothalamus

5 Which of the following is secreted by the kidneys in response to hypoxia?

   a Angiotensin-converting enzyme (ACE)

   b Erythropoietin

   c Leptin

   d Atrial natriuretic peptide (ANP)

   e Thymopoietins

6 Loop diuretics promote diuresis by which of the following mechanisms?

a H^+/K^+ transporter inhibitor

b Na^+/H^+ pump stimulator

c Carbonic anhydrase inhibitor

d Antidiuretic hormone (ADH) inhibitor

e $Na^+/K^+/2Cl^-$ cotransport inhibitor

7 Loop diuretics most commonly result in which of the following electrolyte abnormalities?

a Hyperkalaemia

b Hypokalaemia

c Hypophosphataemia

d Hypercalcaemia

e All of the above

8 Renin is secreted by the kidney in response to reduced renal perfusion. Which of the following statements best describes the action of this hormone?

a It converts angiotensin I to angiotensin II

b It cleaves angiotensinogen to aldosterone

c It converts angiotensinogen to angiotensin I

d It reduces blood pressure by promoting diuresis

e It causes vasodilation of the glomerulus

9 What is the effect of aldosterone on the effective circulating volume and fluid balance?

   a Aldosterone promotes diuresis and thus reduces the effective circulating volume

   b It results in erythropoietin secretion and thus increases effective circulating volume

   c Aldosterone inhibits reabsorption of sodium and thus promotes water excretion, in order to reduce cardiac preload

   d It acts to decrease preload by directly increasing the collecting-duct water permeability

   e Aldosterone stimulates sodium reabsorption in the collecting duct to increase effective circulating volume

10 Which of the following statements regarding the role of the kidneys in acid–base balance is correct?

   a Respiratory acidosis results in reduction of H^+ secretion by the renal tubules and reduced reabsorption of HCO_3^-

   b The Henderson–Hasselbach equation is used to calculate renal perfusion in disorders of acid–base balance

   c Renal compensation occurs acutely (within hours) in respiratory alkalosis

   d A plasma pH of 7.25 will be compensated by reduced renal HCO_3^- reabsorption

   e Hydrogen ion secretion occurs via H^+ ATPase and the Na^+/H^+ cotransporter

11 Which factor usually prevents glomerular filtration of protein?

a Fenestrated epithelial capillary cells

b Large intracellular gap junctions

c Glomerulonephritis

d Nephrotic syndrome

e All of the above

12 At approximately what urinary volume does an adult initially feel a sensation of bladder fullness?

a 10 mL

b 35 mL

c 100 mL

d 250 mL

e 1 L

13 How much urine would you expect an average 70-kg man to produce in 1 hour?

a 10 mL

b 35 mL

c 100 mL

d 250 mL

e 1 L

14 Which structure is primarily adapted in order to facilitate bladder distensibility?

a The trigone

b Detrusor muscle

c The ureters

d The spermatic cord

e The concentration of urea

15 Approximately what percentage of cardiac output supplies the kidneys?

a 1%

b 10%

c 20%

d 50%

e 80%

16 Following glomerular filtration, the filtrate is similar to plasma except for which of the following?

a The presence of potassium

b The presence of protein

c The absence of protein

d The presence of clotting factors

e The absence of glucose

17 Renal clearance of a solution X can be used to measure the glomerular filtration rate (GFR). Which of the following rules apply in order to measure glomerular filtration rate accurately by this method?

    a Solution X must not be metabolised or synthesised by the kidney

    b Solution X must not be reabsorbed by the kidney

    c Solution X must not be secreted by the kidney

    d Solution X must be freely filtered by the kidney

    e All of the above

18 Which of the following hormones relating to fluid balance is secreted by the lungs?

    a Renin

    b Angiotensin II

    c Angiotensin-converting enzyme (ACE)

    d Aldosterone

    e Antidiuretic hormone (ADH)

19 Which of the following hormones relating to fluid balance is secreted by the adrenal glands?

    a Renin

    b Angiotensin II

    c Angiotensin-converting enzyme (ACE)

    d Aldosterone

    e Antidiuretic hormone (ADH)

20 Which of the following forces promotes glomerular filtration?

a Capillary oncotic pressure

b Urine output

c Hydrostatic pressure from capillaries

d All of the above

e None of the above

21 Which of the following forces opposes glomerular filtration?

a Capillary oncotic pressure

b Urine output

c Hydrostatic pressure from capillaries

d All of the above

e None of the above

22 The production of a small volume of highly concentrated urine may be due to which of the following?

a Dehydration

b Diuretic therapy

c Lack of ADH secretion (e.g. diabetes insipidus)

d All of the above

e None of the above

23 Which of the following situations may lead to the production of a large volume of dilute urine?

a Intravenous fluid rehydration

b Diuretic therapy

c Lack of ADH secretion (e.g. diabetes insipidus)

d All of the above

e None of the above

24 Despite increases in blood pressure, the glomerular filtration rate (GFR) of the kidneys remains relatively constant. By which of the following mechanisms do the kidneys maintain a steady GFR?

a Reduction in cardiac output

b Systemic vasodilatation

c Secretion of aldosterone

d Autoregulation

e Increase in GFR

25 Following glomerular filtration, the filtrate passes through the proximal tubule and on to the loop of Henle. Approximately what percentage of the filtrate is reabsorbed at the loop of Henle?

a None

b 1%

c 20%

d 80%

e 100%

26 Which of the following is an obstructive cause of renal failure?

a Dehydration

b Hypovolaemia

c Glomerulonephritis

d Acute tubular necrosis

e Benign prostatic hyperplasia (enlargement of the prostate)

Extended matching questions

Theme: Acid–base balance and the kidneys

a Hyperventilation

b Diabetic ketoacidosis

c Depression

d Bulimia

e Opiate overdose

f Aspirin overdose

g Hyperthyroidism

h Increased anion gap

i Decreased anion gap

j Normal anion gap

For each of the following questions, select the most appropriate answer from the list of options above. Each option may be used once, more than once or not at all.

1 Respiratory compensation of metabolic acidosis

2 A cause of metabolic alkalosis

3 A cause of respiratory alkalosis

4 The effect of lactic acidosis on the anion gap

5 The effect of renal tubular acidosis on the anion gap

Theme: The renin–angiotensin–aldosterone axis

a Renin

b Aldosterone

c Cortisol

d Atrial natriuretic peptide (ANP)

e Vasodilatation

f Vasoconstriction

g No effect

h 1%

i 10%

j 15%

k 50%

l 85%

For each of the following questions, select the most appropriate answer from the list of options above. Each option may be used once, more than once or not at all.

1 A reduction in extracellular volume promotes the release of which substance from the kidney?

2 What is the effect of angiotensin II on renal vasculature?

3 Which hormone antagonises the renin–angiotensin–aldosterone axis?

4 What percentage reduction of extracellular fluid would stimulate antidiuretic hormone (ADH) release?

5 What percentage increase in osmolarity would stimulate ADH release?

Theme: Renal transplantation

a   Pruritus (itch)

b   Arteriovenous (AV) fistula

c   Systemic lupus erythematosus (SLE)

d   Renal cell carcinoma

e   Vasopressin

f   Diabetes mellitus

g   Unilateral functioning kidney

h   Ciclosporin

i   Amoxicillin

j   Insulin

k   Loin

l   Iliac fossa

m   Immunosuppressants

For each of the following questions, select the most appropriate answer from the list of options above. Each option may be used once, more than once or not at all.

1   Renal transplantation incurs many risks. Which factor makes a patient more susceptible to infection?

2   Which examination finding would suggest previous renal replacement therapy?

3   The commonest cause of chronic renal failure in the UK

4   Name a drug given to transplant recipients

5   At which site is the transplanted kidney inserted?

Theme: Monitoring and maintaining fluid balance

a Autoregulation

b Filtration

c Reabsorption

d Glomerular filtration rate

e Cardiac output

f Juxtaglomerular apparatus

g Medulla

h Zona glomerulosa

i Posterior pituitary gland

j Anterior pituitary gland

k Hypothalamus

For each of the following questions, select the most appropriate answer from the list of options above. Each option may be used once, more than once or not at all.

1 The area which detects changes in osmolarity

2 The region responsible for antidiuretic hormone (ADH) secretion

3 The process by which glomerular filtration rate is held steady in situations of increased blood pressure

4 The area which is responsible for the secretion of renin

5 A product of stroke volume and heart rate

Answers

Section 1: Neuromuscular physiology

1 d

The autonomic nervous system utilises two primary neurotransmitters: acetylcholine and noradrenaline. The preganglionic neurons of both the sympathetic and parasympathetic systems are cholinergic, while postganglionic sympathetic neurons secrete both acetylcholine and noradrenaline.

2 e

Stimulation of the parasympathetic nervous system is responsible for contraction of the sphincter muscles of the iris, resulting in pupillary constriction. The sympathetic system does the opposite. Always remember the saying 'Eyes wide with fright'.

3 d

Stimulation of the β_2-adrenergic receptors results in actions as diverse as vasodilatation of the skeletal muscle vasculature to relaxation of the uterus and glycogenesis. Drugs acting as agonists at the β_2-receptors can be delivered as inhalers to facilitate bronchodilation, e.g. salbutamol and terbutaline, in respiratory disease, such as asthma.

4 b

The nicotinic cholinergic receptors facilitate transmission between the pre- and postganglionic neurons of both branches of the autonomic nervous system, as well as at the neuromuscular junction.

5 a

Neostigmine is an acetylcholinesterase inhibitor, which blocks the breakdown of acetylcholine, thus prolonging its action. Acetylcholinesterase inhibitors can be used at the neuromuscular junction (NMJ) to enhance transmission in myasthenia gravis, an autoimmune disease resulting in NMJ-receptor blockade.

6 a

The oligodendrocytes form the myelin sheath in the central nervous system. In contrast to the Schwann cells of the peripheral nervous system, they can insulate up to 50 axons at once. The myelinated fibres of the CNS form the 'white matter'.

7 b

Schwann cells surround the nerve fibres to form the myelin sheath of the peripheral nervous system. Myelin creates an electrical insulator around the fibre and allows a much faster rate of conduction than the unmyelinated axons. The fastest myelinating conducting fibres are Aα, which innervate skeletal muscle and Aγ.

8 d

The blood–brain barrier is a protective mechanism, preventing the brain capillary content from entering the neuronal and extracellular tissue. It is composed of tight junctions of the capillary endothelium, astrocytes and the basal lamina. The blood–brain barrier is selectively permeable to glucose, amino acids and electrolytes, and readily permeable to fat-soluble molecules. Large plasma proteins cannot permeate the barrier.

9 b

Hyoscine is a muscarinic antagonist used in palliative care to reduce salivation and respiratory secretions. Tricyclic antidepressants have an antagonistic effect at muscarinic receptors and thus exhibit anti-muscarinic side-effects which include urinary retention, increased intraocular pressure (thus worsening of glaucoma) and constipation.

10 d

The basal ganglia are made up of the caudate nucleus, putamen and globus pallidus. The role of the basal ganglia in motor control is still not fully understood. Basal ganglia dysfunction results in motor disorders, such as Parkinson's and Huntington's disease.

11 b

Gamma-aminobutyric acid (GABA) is the major inhibitory transmitter of the central nervous system. It plays a vital role in presynaptic inhibition at axonal synapses.

12 b

The parotid gland is supplied by the parasympathetic branch of the glossopharyngeal nerve. The preganglionic parasympathetic fibres originate in the inferior salivatory nucleus. These neurons synapse with postganglionic neurons in the otic ganglion.

13 c

The nigrostriatal pathway runs from the pars compacta of the substantia nigra and exhibits both inhibitory and excitatory effects upon striatal neurons.

14 a

Long-term potentiation (LTP) is a persistent change in synaptic strength mediated by the N-methyl-D-aspartate (NMDA) receptor, which acts as a calcium channel, blocked at rest by Mg^{2+}.

15 e

The sensory modalities of temperature and pain travel together in the spinothalamic white-matter tract of the spinal cord. The tract carries second-order neurons which decussate to the contralateral side of the cord via the ventral white commissure.

16 b

The resting membrane potential is maintained by the Na^+/K^+ ATPase pump. It establishes a high extracellular Na^+ and a high intracellular K^+ by transporting at a ratio of 3 Na^+ to 2 K^+. Depolarisation of the cell membrane and influx of Na^+ into the cell results in initiation of the action potential.

17 e

In a myopic eye, the image of a near object will fall on the retina, but those from further distances fall in front of the retina. A concave lens diverges the light so that the image focuses directly onto the retina, thus correcting the defect.

18 e

The facial nerve supplies the muscles of facial expression, while the muscles of mastication (pterygoids, temporalis and masseter) are supplied by the motor branch of the trigeminal nerve.

19 a

Striking the patella tendon with a tendon hammer causes passive stretching of the muscle which is detected by muscle spindles. Afferent signals from the muscle spindles travel via the Ia nerve. The α-motor neuron then carries efferent signals to facilitate contraction of the rectus femoris, resulting in extension of the knee. Tendon reflexes form an integral part of the nervous-system examination. Exaggerated reflexes occur in upper motor neuron (UMN) lesions, while diminished reflexes occur in lower motor neuron (LMN) lesions.

20 c

Anaerobic respiration from glycolysis produces ATP, with lactic acid as a by-product. Accumulation of lactic acid in the muscle is painful, resulting in the use of anaerobic respiration for only short, fast, powerful muscle activity.

21 c

Fast glycolytic fibres function to provide quick, fast and powerful contractions. ATP synthesis occurs via anaerobic metabolism, resulting in the accumulation of lactic acid and thus a fast rate of fatigability. Being composed of anaerobic cells, the fibres have less myoglobin (and so appear white or pale) and have only few mitochondria.

22 b

Slow fibres are also known as 'red muscle' because of their high levels of myoglobin. They have a large number of mitochondria, for high levels of oxidative metabolism. Fast fibres, or white muscle, are larger and have large amounts of glycolytic enzymes for the rapid release of energy. Fast fibres are used for short-acting, powerful contraction.

23 c

In periods of starvation, muscle proteins can be utilized for gluconeogenesis. Gluconeogenesis is the formation of glucose from non-carbohydrate precursors. Amino acids (mainly alanine) from muscle proteins provide the source of pyruvate for gluconeogenesis in the liver:

$$2 \text{ pyruvate} + 2 \text{ NADH} + 4 \text{ ATP} + 2 \text{ GTP} \rightarrow \text{glucose} + 2 \text{ NAD}^+ + 4 \text{ ADP} + 2 \text{ GDP} + 6 \text{ P}_i$$

24 e

Muscle contraction is dependent on various factors, including initial stretch of the muscle. This is described by the length–tension relationship: increasing the initial stretch of the muscle fibres causes an increased force of contraction, up to an optimum muscle length, at which overlap between actin and myosin is optimal. Beyond this optimal length, the two filaments are pulled too far apart and the actin–myosin overlap is inadequate to produce a strong contraction.

25 b

The contraction of smooth muscle is slow, to allow for controlled, sustained movement, requiring a lower rate of energy consumption. The action potentials have a slower, longer-lasting upstroke, as voltage-gated calcium channels are activated and calcium is released from stores in the sarcoplasmic reticulum. Calcium ions bind to calmodulin and via myosin light-chain (MLC) kinase result in contraction.

26 e

Tetany occurs when there is a sequence of high-frequency quick-fire action potentials, whereby the second fires before the muscle fibre has relaxed from the first. Tetany can occur in states of severe hypocalcaemia.

Theme: Physiology of skeletal, cardiac and smooth muscle

1 e

2 i

3 b

4 g

5 a

1 e

Skeletal or striated muscle is comprised of fast and slow fibres, which are adapted for different functions. Slow fibres are adapted for prolonged muscle contraction, e.g. postural muscles, while fast fibres are used for short-acting, powerful muscle contractions. Slow fibres are known as red muscle because of their high levels of myoglobin. They have a large number of mitochondria for high levels of oxidative metabolism. Fast fibres, or white muscle, are larger and have a high content of glycolytic enzymes for rapid energy release.

2 i

The motor neuron and muscle fibre form the neuromuscular junction (NMJ). Initiation of a presynaptic action potential results in the influx of calcium ions into the presynaptic cell. Acetylcholine-containing (ACh) vesicles diffuse across the cell and fuse with the neural membrane, releasing ACh into the cleft. Nicotinic ACh receptors on the postsynaptic membrane are activated and result in a positively charged influx of Na^+ into the postsynaptic cell – the end-plate potential. If this potential change is above a specific threshold, an action potential is fired. ACh is broken down by acetylcholinesterase in the synaptic cleft, and this terminates the response.

3 b

Smooth muscle can be divided into two main types: multi-unit, where fibres can contract independently of one another (e.g. ciliary muscle of the iris), and single-unit, whereby muscle fibres contract as a single unit (e.g. visceral muscle of the gut wall). Unlike skeletal muscle, smooth muscle is not organised in a striated fashion but myosin filaments are interspersed amongst the actin filaments. The cycling of cross-bridges between the two filaments is much slower in smooth muscle than skeletal, which allows for prolonged tonic contraction.

4 g

Muscle contraction occurs by cross-bridge formation between thin and thick filaments. Thin filaments are made of actin, while the thick are comprised mainly of myosin. Thick and thin filaments are arranged so that they interdigitate with one another. Muscle contraction is brought about by thin filaments moving over the thick filaments via ATP-dependent cross-bridge formation in a 'walk-along' mechanism.

5 a

Coronary artery occlusion can result from the rupture of an atherosclerotic plaque and thrombus formation. The area of cardiac muscle which is not getting adequately perfused will become ischaemic, and as a result necrosis and infarction occurs. Along with the history, examination and 'cardiac-marker' blood tests, the electrocardiogram (ECG) can diagnose a myocardial infarction (MI). Changes in the ECG include elevation of the ST segment, inversion of T waves and the presence of 'pathological' Q waves.

Theme: Neurotransmitters

1 a

2 d

3 a

4 e

5 b

1 a

The neuromuscular junction (NMJ) is the interface at which an excitatory neuronal impulse can result in contraction of a muscle. Acetylcholine is released into the synaptic cleft at the NMJ in response to neuronal excitation and binds to nicotinic receptors on the muscle fibre.

2 d

The major inhibitory neurotransmitter in the central nervous system is gamma-aminobutyric acid (GABA). Activation of GABA receptors results in an influx of Cl^- ions, resulting in a more negative potential difference across the cell membrane, and thus hyperpolarisation.

3 a

Both the sympathetic and parasympathetic branches of the autonomic nervous system utilise acetylcholine as the neurotransmitter at the preganglionic neuron, which binds to postganglionic nicotinic receptors (as occurs at the NMJ).

4 e

Nicotinic receptors exist on the postsynaptic neurons of both parasympathetic and sympathetic systems.

5 b

Levodopa is a precursor of the neurotransmitter dopamine, and thus can be used in the management of Parkinson's disease, in which there is a deficiency of dopaminergic neurons in the nigrostriatal pathway of the basal ganglia. L-Dopa must be given alongside a decarboxylase inhibitor to prevent peripheral breakdown of the precursor drug and promote its central effect.

Theme: The musculoskeletal system

1 j

2 f

3 d

4 b

5 h

1 j

Striated or skeletal muscle is comprised of myofibrils, which are divided into sarcomeres. Muscle contraction is brought about by the action of two filaments – myosin and actin. Myosin filaments are thicker than actin filaments, and the two are arranged so they inter-digitate with one another. The degree of overlap determines the force of contraction.

2 f

Skeletal muscle is organised in a striated fashion, with darker and lighter bands. The dark bands are due to overlap of the myosin and actin filaments, while the lighter bands only contain actin. Contraction takes place via ATP-dependent cross-bridge formation in the follow-ing stages:

- ATP binds to the myosin head group
- Actin dissociates from myosin
- ATP → ADP + Pi (orthophosphate)
- The myosin head group pivots so that it is at a 90-degree angle with actin filaments
- The myosin head group binds to actin
- The release of Pi causes the 'power stroke', by which the myosin head pivots through 45 degrees, moving actin with respect to the myosin
- ADP is released to complete and restart the cycle

3 d

Ligaments classically describe the connective tissue structure that joins bone to bone, while tendons attach bone to muscle. Simple examples include the inguinal ligament, which connects the anterior superior iliac spine (ASIS) and the pubic tubercle, and the quadriceps tendon, which attaches the hip flexor (quadriceps femoris) to the patella.

4 b

Elbow flexion is brought about by contraction of the biceps brachii, brachioradialis, brachialis and coracobrachialis. They are therefore the elbow-flexion 'agonists'. The 'antagonist', the triceps, works to oppose this movement, and thus triceps contraction results in elbow extension.

5 h

Enthesitis is the inflammation of the site of attachment of tendon or ligaments. A common condition predisposing to enthesitis is ankylosing spondylitis. Ankylosing spondylitis is a seronegative arthropathy, most commonly occurring in young gentlemen. Sufferers complain of pain and stiffness in the back, which is typically worse in the morning and improves with exercise (cf. osteoarthritis back pain, which is worse at night and after exercise).

Theme: Neuronal transmission

1 a

2 c

3 d

4 b

5 g

1 a

The period following an action potential during which the neuron is 'recovering' and another action potential which cannot be elicited, is the refractory period. This can be divided into relative and absolute refractory periods. The absolute refractory period is the time in which the voltage-gated Na^+ channels 'recover' and there are insufficient activated channels to initiate an action potential. The relative refractory period occurs at a time of slow K^+ channel closure, in which an action potential could be elicited, but would require a greater electrical stimulus.

2 c

The potential difference between the extracellular and intracellular components of the cell membrane is its membrane potential. At equilibrium, there is no net movement of ions from one side of the membrane to the other, i.e. the chemical and electrical gradients are equal but opposite. The action of the Na^+/K^+ ATPase pump results in a high extracellular concentration of sodium and high intracellular potassium. As the cell membrane is more permeable to potassium than other ions, potassium ions move down their concentration gradient out of the cell, resulting in a negative intracellular side compared with the outside of the membrane. The resting potential in a mammalian cell is approximately $-70\,mV$.

3 d

An action potential results from the displacement of the electrical current across the cell membrane by changes in ion permeability across the membrane. A chemical or physical stimulus results in a slight increase in the resting membrane potential. When the membrane potential reaches a threshold, voltage-gated Na^+ channels open, so that sodium ions enter the cell down the concentration gradient (from an area of high concentration outside the cell to lower inside the cell). The normally negative membrane potential therefore reverses and becomes positive, i.e. depolarisation (as there are now more positive ions inside the cell relative to the outside).

4 b

The absolute refractory period occurs following the action potential when Na^+ channels are inactivated and there are insufficient Na^+ channels active to allow sodium influx. This prevents a further action potential.

5 g

Following the action potential, in which the membrane potential is positive, Na^+ channels become inactive and voltage-gated potassium channels allow for an efflux of K^+, thus stabilising the membrane potential, i.e. repolarisation.

Section 2: Cardiovascular and respiratory physiology

1 b

The action of noradrenaline on vascular $\alpha 1$ receptors results in vaso-constriction of the vessel. Sympathetic activation of peripheral blood vessels results in constriction and thus diversion of the blood supply away from the peripheries to the vital organs, giving an appearance of pallor.

2 e

Cardiac output is a product of heart rate and stroke volume, thus a faster heart rate results in an increased cardiac output.

3 b

The Frank–Starling law states that the force of cardiac myocyte contraction is related to the volume of blood returning to the heart: the end-diastolic volume (or preload). Much like skeletal muscle, the force of myocyte contraction in the heart is determined by muscle fibre length. At optimal overlap of actin and myosin filaments, and thus optimal length, contraction is greatest. In the heart, this length is determined by the volume of blood and distension of the ventricle prior to contraction (i.e. the preload).

4   d

After ascent to levels of higher altitude, the body's partial pressure of oxygen (pO_2) decreases. Acclimatisation is the process by which the body adapts to the lower concentration of environmental oxygen. Erythropoietin is produced by the kidneys in order to stimulate erythrocytic production in the bone marrow and thus increase the oxygen-carrying capacity of the blood.

5   b

Electrical activity in the heart travels from the cardiac 'intrinsic pacemaker', the sinoatrial node (SAN) in the right atrium. From the SAN, electrical impulses are carried to the atrioventricular node (AVN), which allows the passage of the signal between the atria and ventricles. The impulse is then transmitted down the bundle of His, which in turn divides into right and left bundles. The bundles pass along the right and left side of the interventricular septum. If one of the bundles is blocked, that bundle no longer conducts an impulse, and the two ventricles do not receive an impulse simultaneously.

6   a

Heart rate is normally determined by the sinoatrial node in the right atrium. It has the highest frequency of activity, and therefore overrides other potential ectopic areas.

7   e

In a state of third-degree or complete heart block, there is no relationship between atrial and ventricular contraction. The atria continue to contract at a rate determined by the sinoatrial node, while the ventricles contract independently. A cardiac pacemaker can be used in this situation.

8   e

Atrial fibrillation (AF) is an irregularly irregular heart rhythm which predisposes to thromboembolic events, such as cerebrovascular disease. Patients with AF should be classified as to their thromboembolic risk and anticoagulated with aspirin or warfarin accordingly (ensuring there are no contraindications). The CHADS-2 score can be calculated in order to determine this (see below). A patient scoring 1 can be managed with aspirin or warfarin, while a score of 2 or above indicates that warfarin may be the most appropriate choice.

CHADS-2
- **C**ardiac failure – impaired left ventricular function, or clinical evidence of failure or valvular disease
- **H**ypertension
- **A**ge >65
- **D**iabetes mellitus
- **S**troke – previous stroke, TIA or thromboembolic event (scores **2**)

9 c

The ECG is comprised of P, Q, R, S and T waves. Put very simply, these are derived from the following.

Wave on ECG	Corresponding element of cardiac cycle
p	Atrial depolarisation
QRS	Ventricular depolarisation
T	Ventricular repolarisation

10 b

The rate of depolarisation at the sinoatrial node and thus heart rate can be manipulated by several different means. The autonomic nervous system affects the rate of contraction. Sympathetic activity increases heart rate by reducing the delay in depolarisation and also increasing the speed of conduction through the atrioventricular node.

11 b

Stenosis or narrowing of the aortic valve can occur secondary to atherosclerotic disease, or may be a primary congenital malformation. Outflow obstruction of the left ventricle secondary to aortic stenosis results in hypertrophy of the muscle, as the left ventricle has to pump harder to force blood through the narrowed valve.

12 e

The ejection fraction is a good measure of cardiac function and is approximately 60% in a normal heart.

13 e

Atherosclerosis is accountable for a wide range of vascular disease, e.g. myocardial infarction and stroke. There are a number of risk factors predisposing to the development of atherosclerotic disease, some modifiable and others not so.

Modifiable risk factors	Non-modifiable risk factors
Hypertension	Family history
Hyperlipidaemia (non-familial)	Age
Diabetic control (modifiable to a certain extent)	Male gender (vs. women premenopause)
Sedentary lifestyle	Homocystinuria
Obesity	Diabetes mellitus
Smoking	Familial hyperlipidaemia
Alcohol intake	

14 c

On standing up, blood pools into the lower limbs, due to the effects of gravity. This results in a reduction in preload and thus a reduction in stroke volume and cardiac output (Frank–Starling law). Subsequently, this is detected by baroreceptors, resulting in activation of the sympathetic system. The sympathetic system initiates an increase in heart rate and peripheral vasoconstriction, thus normalising preload and cardiac output.

15 b

Hypoventilation, which may be secondary to drugs or neuromuscular disease, results in a reduction in the offloading of CO_2 from the blood. A rise in CO_2 results in decreased pH and acidosis.

$$pH = 6.1 + \frac{\log HCO_3^-}{0.03 \times pCO_2}$$

16 b

The residual volume of the lungs is that following a maximal expiration. This mechanism works to prevent collapse of the alveoli following expiration.

17 d

Poiseuille's law gives us the equation for resistance. In keeping with the above equation, flow rate of the airways is highly dependent (to the power 4) on the radius of the tube. Bronchoconstriction secondary to asthma and anaphylaxis therefore severely reduces flow through the airways.

18 c

The autoregulatory mechanism of the lungs allows for maximal transfer of oxygen. At low levels of oxygen (i.e. a pulmonary region with poor ventilation), the pulmonary vasculature constricts so that the blood bypasses this area to favour the oxygen-rich alveoli.

19 e

Surfactant is synthesised from fatty acids in the lung. Areas of poorly perfused lung cannot extract fatty acids from the blood, and thus surfactant may be depleted.

20 c

Surfactant is a detergent-like complex which reduces the work of breathing required to expand the lung by reducing the alveolar surface tension and increasing its compliance. Surfactant is produced late in the third trimester of pregnancy, and premature babies (<34–36 weeks) may lack surfactant and develop respiratory distress syndrome, which can be fatal.

21 e

Public knowledge of the detrimental effects of smoking and its link to respiratory problems, cancers, cardiovascular disease and stroke is now widespread. Chronic obstructive airways disease occurs secondary to inflammation of the airways, in response to permanent damage from smoking. The lifetime risk of a smoker developing lung cancer is 15–30 times higher than that of a non-smoker.

22 e

Terbutaline and salbutamol are β_2-agonists which result in bronchodilation. They may be 'as required' inhalers for patients with mild asthma, or may be given via a nebuliser with high-flow oxygen in severe acute asthma attacks.

23 a

The haemoglobin–oxygen dissociation curve is shifted to the right in environments with raised carbon dioxide, 2,3-diphosphoglycerate (2,3-DPG), H^+ and temperature. This allows oxygen to be offloaded from the blood to the respiring tissues more readily. For example, an increase in 2,3-DPG (a by-product of red cell metabolism) results in a shift of the curve to the right, and thus oxygen is more readily available to the tissues.

24 c

$$CO_2 + H_20 \leftrightarrow H_2CO_3 \leftrightarrow H^+ + HCO_3^-$$

Carbon dioxide is taken up from the tissues into the blood and combines with water to form carbonic acid, which then dissociates to H^+ and HCO_3^-. This reaction is catalysed by carbonic anhydrase, which is found in erythrocytes. The bicarbonate ion is transferred out of the erythrocyte for chloride, and the remaining hydrogen ions are buffered by haemoglobin in the erythrocyte.

25 c

The blood–brain barrier is permeable to carbon dioxide, and it is the arterial CO_2 which plays the greatest role in the regulation of respiratory rate. An increase in cerebrospinal fluid (CSF) CO_2 results in a decreased pH (as per the Henderson–Hasselbach equation). The pH of CSF determines the extracellular pH, which is then detected by central chemoreceptors, and the rate of respiration increases accordingly.

26 a

An increase in temperature, along with increases in carbon dioxide, H^+ and 2,3-diphosphoglycerate (2,3-DPG), cause the haemoglobin–oxygen curve to shift to the right. You may notice that these are all features of metabolic activity. When the tissue is working harder (e.g. exercising muscle), by shifting of the $Hb–O_2$ curve to the right, oxygen can be offloaded from the haemoglobin molecule more readily at a given pO_2, thus providing available oxygen to the respiring tissue. Increasing the respiratory rate allows more oxygen to be available and offloads carbon dioxide built up during increased respiration. In animals, an increased respiratory rate may be noticed as 'panting' when the animal is hot.

Theme: Cardiovascular pharmacology

1 a

2 b

3 a

4 a

5 d

1 a

Digoxin is a cardiac glycoside used in atrial fibrillation, atrial flutter and in heart failure. It acts on the Na^+/K^+ ATPase pump to reduce its activity, thus increasing intracellular Na^+, and therefore Ca^{2+}. The overall effect is to increase the time between action potentials and thus decrease the heart rate.

2 b

Noradrenaline is an inotropic agent which acts at the adrenergic receptors. An inotrope is a drug that increases the rate of cardiac contraction, and thus noradrenaline is used in the intensive care setting in circulatory failure and refractory hypotension.

3 a

Digoxin derives from the foxglove plant *Digitalis lanata*. It is used for rate control in atrial fibrillation and atrial flutter. Its mildly positive inotropic properties give it a role in congestive cardiac failure.

4 a

Examiners occasionally like to confuse candidates by selecting the same answer a few times in one extended matching question; don't be put off by this! Digoxin has mildly positive inotropic properties (i.e. mildly strengthens the force of contractility), in addition to its negative chronotropic activity. From the Greek *chrono*, meaning time, a negative chronotrope is one which slows down the heart rate, while a positive chronotrope (e.g. atropine) increases the heart rate.

5 d

Beta blockers are widely used negative chronotropes. They are used in rate control of tachyarrythmias and still have a role in the management of poorly controlled hypertension. They also act as vasoconstrictors, resulting in a number of side effects associated with their use, including cold extremities and erectile dysfunction.

Theme: Physiology and structure of the heart

1 i

2 e

3 g

4 f

5 e

1 i

Deoxygenated blood containing high pCO_2 from the respiring body tissues returns to the heart in order to be sent to take part in gaseous exchange at the alveoli. Venous blood collects in the vena cavae (superior and inferior branches) and returns to the right atrium. The right ventricle then pumps the venous blood to the lungs via the pulmonary artery, where it can undergo gaseous exchange.

2 e

The intrinsic pacemaker of the heart, the sinoatrial node (SAN) is situated in the posterior wall of the right atrium. Cells of the SAN regularly spontaneously depolarise to dictate the rate of cardiac contraction.

3 g

The bundle of His transmits depolarisation across the annulus fibrosus and the interventricular septum. It splits in to right, left, anterior and posterior bundles, and they transmit the depolarisation to the Purkinje fibres, resulting in coordinated contraction of the ventricles.

4 f

The atria and ventricles are well insulated to prevent passage of the electrical impulse between the two. The atrioventricular node serves this function, allowing an adequate delay between atria and ventricular contraction.

5 e

In order to control the heart rate and override any potential ectopic pacemaker areas, the sinoatrial node (SAN) must have the highest spontaneous rate of depolarisation. The frequency of depolarisation at the SAN dictates the heart rate.

Theme: Reversible causes of cardiac arrest

1 e

2 a

3 g

4 b

5 c

1 e

This question is a little tricky, as you may be tempted to answer hypovolaemia. An extensive bleed would indeed lead to hypovolaemia, but the principal cause of the arrest in this case would be hypoxia, due to hypoperfusion of the cardiac tissue with oxygenated haemoglobin. It is the oxygen from the blood which the heart principally needs.

2 a

A tension pneumothorax results in classical examination findings. There will be decreased breath sounds and hyperresonance to percussion on the affected side. The whole mediastinum shifts away from the pneumothorax, and the trachea can be palpated to confirm this.

3 g

Metabolic disturbance, particularly hyperkalaemia, can result in arrhythmias and ultimately cardiac arrest. The gentleman in question is taking several medicines known to increase serum potassium.

4 b

One must not forget the possibility of toxins in a cardiac arrest situation. Several illegal drugs and prescribed medicines (if taken incorrectly) can result in cardiac arrest. Amphetamines and other drugs of abuse can lead to arrest in a young, previously healthy individual.

5 c

The most common cause of a cardiac arrest is thromboembolism. This includes arrest resulting from a large myocardial infarction or from a massive pulmonary embolism.

Don't forget the **four Ts** and **four Hs** of cardiac arrest:

- **T**hromboembolism
- **T**oxins
- **T**amponade
- **T**ension pneumothorax
- **H**ypoxia
- **H**ypovolaemia
- **H**yperkalaemia (and other electrolyte disturbance)
- **H**ypothermia

Theme: Respiratory physiology

1 b

2 a

3 h

4 c

5 d

1 b

The tidal volume is the volume of air inspired and expired during normal relaxed breathing. It is approximately 500 mL in the average adult.

2 a

Dead space implies the regions of the respiratory system which do not directly take part in gaseous exchange, e.g. the airways. It is approximately 150 mL.

3 h

Hyperventilation is the process of increasing respiratory rate, and thus blowing off carbon dioxide more quickly. A reduction in CO_2 results in a decrease in hydrogen ions, and thus makes the pH more alkalotic. As the alkalosis is occurring from respiratory means, rather than metabolic, the alkalosis is respiratory in nature, hence respiratory alkalosis.

4 c

To compensate for a decrease in pH, the respiratory system increases ventilatory rate. This allows for the removal of CO_2, and thus brings up the pH.

$$pH = 6.1 + \frac{\log HCO_3^-}{0.03 \times pCO_2}$$

It may seem difficult to try and remember the effects of CO_2 and pH with the above equation, so just think of CO_2 as an acid to serum. When breathing is slowed down and CO_2 accumulates, the body becomes more acidic, and when breathing rate increases, CO_2 decreases and the body becomes more alkali.

5 d

An alkalotic environment can be compensated for by reducing the rate of respiration. Accumulation of CO_2 results in an increase in H^+, and thus reduced pH.

Remember:

- H **I** gh CO_2 = Ac **I** dosis
- **L** ow CO_2 = A **L** ka **L** osis

Section 3: Gastrointestinal and metabolism

1 e

Atrial natriuretic peptide (ANP) is produced by the cardiac myocytes of the atria in response to increased venous return. It acts to stimulate salt and water excretion. The remaining four hormones all act as part of the gastrointestinal and hepatobiliary systems. Cholecystokinin augments gall bladder contraction and sphincter relaxation in response to fat in the duodenum; secretin controls duodenal secretions; gastric inhibitory peptide plays a role in fatty acid metabolism and gastrin stimulates gastric acid secretion.

2 c

Intrinsic factor is required for vitamin B_{12} absorption and is secreted from parietal cells. Antibodies against intrinsic factor, or against the parietal cells themselves, result in vitamin B_{12} deficiency and a macrocytosis, a condition called pernicious anaemia.

3 a

Hepatic detoxification of alcohol requires the presence of ethanol dehydrogenase, which catalyses the above reaction. The product of the reaction, acetate can be conjugated and forms fatty acids, the pathogenesis behind obesity and fatty liver disease in alcoholics.

4 b

Synthetic function of the liver is best assessed by the albumin level. The transaminase enzymes, AST and ALT indicate intrinsic hepatic function, while ALP and γGT are raised in biliary obstruction.

5 c

Chief cells of the stomach are responsible for the secretion of pepsinogen, which is activated in response to an acidic environment. Activated pepsin plays a role in the digestion of proteins.

6 a

Cholecystokinin is responsible for the release of bile from the gall bladder and is stimulated by the presence of fat in the duodenum. Bile emulsifies dietary fats, allowing for digestion and absorption.

7 e

The liver is responsible for the synthesis of clotting factors, many of which are vitamin K–dependent. A deficiency of vitamin K can therefore lead to bleeding complications and is given to newborn babies to prevent haemolytic disease. Factors VII, IX and X and prothrombin are all vitamin K–dependent.

8 d

Ileus is paralysis of the bowel, which can occur temporarily following bowel surgery. Potassium is important for the function of peristalsis, and hypokalaemia is commonly found in patients suffering with ileus.

9 d

This is a slightly tricky question. When bowel complications necessitate surgical resection, there may be insufficient length left for adequate nutritional absorption. The other three options in the question all use the enteric route, and thus still require a sufficient length of intestine to facilitate absorption. Total parenteral nutrition involves administering the nutrients directly into the bloodstream (via a central venous catheter), thus bypassing the bowel entirely.

10 e

Intestinal obstruction prevents the passage of bowel content from anywhere between the stomach and the rectum. Complete obstruction will lead to absolute constipation (i.e. neither flatus nor faeces passed). Overflow diarrhoea can become a problem in chronic constipation, but when there is complete obstruction, absolute constipation will occur.

11 b

H^+/K^+ ATPase on the luminal membrane of the parietal cell results in the movement of hydrogen ions into the gastric lumen. The presence of food in the stomach results in an increase in gastric acid secretion. Approximately 2 L of hydrochloric acid is secreted each day. Hydrochloric acid facilitates the action and formation of enzymes such as pepsin, which augments protein digestion.

12 b

Pancreatic β-cells are responsible for insulin secretion. Insulin is secreted in response to hyperglycaemia following a meal and converts blood glucose into glycogen stores.

13 e

Gastric secretions enable digestion. Stimulation of secretions occur from the very thought of food! Taste and smell stimulate vagal activity, which subsequently promotes secretion. Similarly, gastric distension initiates vagal activity, and protein digestion results in G-cell secretion of gastrin.

14 e

Helicobacter pylori, NSAIDs, aspirin and alcohol can all damage the gastric mucosa and predispose to gastric erosion and peptic ulcers. Somatostatin, secreted by the endocrine D cells, reduces gastric acid production. *H. pylori* inhibits somatostatin and is a common cause of peptic ulcer disease. Patients with ulcers can be tested for the presence of *H. pylori* and eradication therapy given to help prevent recurrence.

15 b

Patients who have had a period of poor nutrition are at risk of refeeding syndrome with the reintroduction of food. The presence of glucose results in insulin secretion, which drives fat, protein and glycogen synthesis. These processes also require electrolytes, including magnesium and phosphate. This further depletes a sparse supply, and can lead to fatal hypophosphataemia.

16 b

The proton-pump inhibitors, e.g. lansoprazole, omeprazole, pantoprazole, act on the H^+/K^+ ATPase pump to reduce gastric acid secretion. They provide symptomatic relief in reflux disease, help in the prevention of peptic ulcer disease and reduce small-bowel stoma outputs by reducing gastric secretions.

17 e

The spleen is a retroperitoneal structure of the abdomen. It has a reticuloendothelial role. Due to its vast blood supply, abdominal trauma can be life-threatening, due to haemorrhage from splenic rupture. These cases necessitate life-saving splenectomy. Post-operatively, without the immunoprotection of the spleen, patients need vaccinating against meningococcal and pneumococcal species and will need lifelong antibiotic prophylaxis.

18 d

Chronic alcoholism can lead to malabsorption due to pancreatic insufficiency. Alcohol abuse leads to destruction of the pancreatic exocrine cells and prevents adequate lipase production. Lipase is required for fat digestion and the absorption of the fat-soluble vitamins A, D, E and K.

19 b

An ileostomy is an opening of the ileum onto the skin surface, whereby bowel content is drained off. Despite the bowel not being in continuity, the same principles apply. Codeine phosphate, an opiate, slows down the gut and thus will reduce the output from a stoma. High fluid output from proximal small-bowel stomas is a complex problem, often resulting in severe dehydration and renal failure; therefore, drugs which slow the bowel, such as loperamide and codeine, prove useful.

20 e

The total iron-binding capacity (TIBC) is high in states of iron deficiency in an attempt to utilise all the available iron. Ferritin is a measure of iron stores, but also a marker of inflammation. It is not a useful indicator of iron levels with coexisting infection or inflammation. The mean corpuscular volume (MCV) is low in states of iron deficiency, but high in vitamin B_{12} and folate-deficiency anaemia.

21 c

Although all of the options are sugars which are commonly present in the diet, glucose is the only monosaccharide in the list of options. Sucrose and lactose are both disaccharides, while starch and glycogen are two examples of polysaccharides.

22 b

Bile is produced in the liver and stored in the gall bladder; therefore, patients who undergo cholecystectomy operations (gall bladder removal) for problematic gallstones do not generally experience problems with fat digestion or absorption post-operatively.

23 d

The motor component of the fifth cranial nerve, the trigeminal nerve, supplies the muscles of chewing (mastication). They are the temporalis, masseter and medial and lateral pterygoids. The three sensory branches of the trigeminal nerve supply facial sensation.

24 d

Vitamins A, D, E and K are all fat-soluble vitamins and require dietary fat for their absorption. Disease processes in which there is fat mal-absorption, e.g. cystic fibrosis, may require vitamin supplementation. Vitamin C is water-soluble and is found in plentiful supply in fresh fruit and vegetables.

25 e

Gastrin is secreted by G cells in response to chemical stimuli in the stomach and rising pH. It targets the parietal cells to stimulate HCl secretion. A low-pH environment inhibits gastrin production, thus completing the negative feedback loop.

26 a

The enterogastric reflex is stimulated by the sympathetic nervous system and reduces gut motility. The parasympathetic system also synapses onto enteric nerves. Remember with regard to the parasympathetic system: 'Rest and digest'.

Theme: Causes of malabsorption

1 f

2 d

3 a

4 c

5 b

1 f

Pernicious anaemia is an autoimmune condition in which there are autoantibodies directed against intrinsic factor or against the parietal cells which produce intrinsic factor, required for the absorption of vitamin B_{12}. Vitamin B_{12} deficiency may present with peripheral neuropathy and results in a megaloblastic anaemia with a raised mean cell volume (MCV).

2 d

Radiotherapy, whether therapeutic or palliative, plays a role in the management of malignancy. Irradiation damage to the bowel can result in malabsorption and may necessitate feeding by other means, e.g. total parenteral nutrition (TPN).

3 a

Cystic fibrosis is an autosomal recessive condition with a genetic change in a region which codes for an epithelial chloride transporter. It is characterised by viscid secretions, resulting in recurrent pulmonary infections as well as pancreatic damage secondary to blockage of the ducts. There is also failure of development of the vas deferens, resulting in male infertility.

4 c

Coeliac disease is a gluten-sensitive enteropathy resulting in villous atrophy and resultant malabsorption. Jejunal biopsy is the gold standard for definitive diagnosis, although an improvement in symptoms with a gluten-free diet gives a clue to the likely cause.

5 b

A blockage of the coeliac or mesenteric vessels can lead to mesenteric ischemia, necessitating life-saving surgery. With widespread ischaemia, a long length of infarcted bowel will be removed, resulting in a short length of gut left for absorption. Short-bowel syndrome occurs when there is less than 200 cm left in situ, with 100 cm or less necessitating parenteral nutrition.

Theme: Minerals and vitamins

1 j

2 h

3 e

4 f

5 i

1 j

The fat-soluble vitamins require dietary fat to be absorbed. They include vitamins A, D, E and K (ADEK). In disease states characterised by fat malabsorption, e.g. chronic pancreatitis, alcoholism and cystic fibrosis, supplementation of the fat-soluble vitamins may be necessary.

2 h

Vitamin C, or ascorbic acid, is a water-soluble vitamin found in fruit and vegetables. It is necessary for collagen synthesis. A lack of dietary vitamin C can result in scurvy, which may present with lethargy, malaise and bleeding of the mucosal membranes.

3 e

Calcium metabolism is controlled by various hormones, including parathyroid hormone (PTH), vitamin D and calcitonin. PTH is secreted from the parathyroid glands in response to hypocalcaemia. It acts to increase renal calcium reabsorption, increases 1α-hydroxylase activity required for the metabolism of vitamin D and increases calcium mobilisation from bone.

4 f

Thiamine (vitamin B_1) is absorbed at low concentrations by active transport in the distal small intestine. Its absorption is inhibited by folic-acid deficiency and alcohol. This explains the common finding of thiamine deficiency in alcoholics, which can lead to Wernicke's encephalopathy, a triad of ophthalmoplegia, ataxia and confusion.

5 i

Vitamin D metabolism occurs via the following pathway and culminates with the formation of its active form, $1,25\text{-}(OH)_2D_3$.

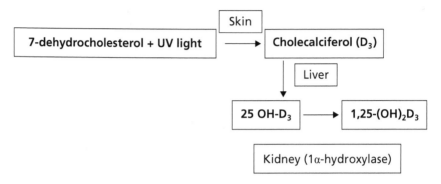

Theme: Functions of the liver

1 g

2 i

3 b

4 a

5 f

1 g

Haemochromatosis may be hereditary or acquired (from frequent transfusions) and results from excess iron levels. Accumulation in the liver, heart and pancreas results in hepatitis, pancreatitis and cardiomyopathy. Regular phlebotomy or iron chelation with desferrioxamine are the mainstay of treatment.

2 i

Portal hypertension is a complication of chronic liver disease and can lead to the formation of dilated vessels – varices. They can rupture and result in massive haematemesis. The patient must be resuscitated and undergo emergency endoscopy in an attempt to stop the bleeding.

3 b

Albumin makes up the majority of plasma protein and plays an important role in fluid distribution and molecular transport. It is a large protein, and deficiency from malnutrition or renal disease results in disruption of extracellular osmolarity and leads to oedema and ascites.

4 a

Ferritin is a marker of the acute-phase response and so is raised in inflammation and infection. It is therefore a poor marker of iron stores in patients with coexisting disease.

5 f

Along with its roles in storage, metabolism and homeostasis, the liver plays an important role in the synthesis of urea from ammonia, which is a toxic compound if left to accumulate.

Theme: The metabolism of glucose

1 h

2 a

3 b

4 i

5 e

1 h

Gluconeogenesis is the formation (*genesis*) of 'new' (*neo*) glucose. The glucose formed from gluconeogenesis may be stored as glycogen or may be used for tissue metabolism in exercise, malnutrition or starvation. Amino acid products of protein breakdown enter the Kreb's cycle, resulting in pyruvate production which is then converted to glucose in the liver. Body muscle is used as the source of protein in starvation, leading to the typical wasted and emaciated appearance of malnourished individuals.

2 a

Glycogenolysis is the breakdown of glycogen to release glucose, catalysed by glycogen phosphorylase.

3 b

Glycogenesis is the process of glycogen synthesis from glucose.

4 i

Glycolysis is the cytoplasmic process by which pyruvate is metabolised from glucose in order to enter the Kreb's cycle.

5 e

Glucagon is a peptide hormone released from α-cells of the pancreas in response to hypoglycaemia. Very high levels of glucagon indicate severe hypoglycaemia, and thus at high levels it also stimulates lipolysis and ketogenesis.

Section 4: Endocrinology and reproduction

1 c

The menstrual cycle is controlled by the hypothalamic–pituitary–ovarian axis. Gonadotrophin-releasing hormone (GnRH) is released from the hypothalamus, which stimulates the anterior pituitary to secrete follicle-stimulating hormone (FSH) and luteinising hormone (LH). The gonadotrophins stimulate follicular growth and ovarian androgen production. Day 1 of the cycle is the first day of menstruation. During the initial (follicular) phase of the cycle, FSH levels are high, promoting growth of the primary follicle. The follicle secretes oestrogen, which stimulates the proliferation of the endometrium. Oestrogen negatively feeds back to reduce gonadotrophin levels. However, above a threshold level of oestrogen, the LH surge occurs. Ovulation is stimulated and occurs within 24 hours.

2 d

During the follicular phase of the menstrual cycle, the primary follicle (developed under the influence of FSH) secretes oestrogen. This induces proliferative changes in the endometrium and at high (above threshold) levels stimulates the LH surge to promote ovulation around day 14 of the cycle.

3 e

The hypothalamic–pituitary–ovarian axis, as shown below, works by positive and negative feedback mechanisms. Ovarian failure results in reduced oestrogen levels. FSH production is inhibited by negative feedback by oestrogen on the pituitary. Low oestrogen levels therefore result in increased FSH.

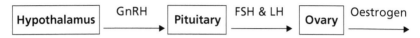

4 e

Oxytocin is secreted from the posterior pituitary and initiates the 'let-down' reflex. This lets milk into the subareolar sinuses to allow excretion from the nipple. It also plays an important role in cervical dilatation and uterine contractions during labour.

5 b

Leydig cells of the testes produce testosterone. Testosterone plays an important role in testicular and prostatic development, as well as the appearance of secondary sexual characteristics and spermatogenesis.

6 e

Surfactant is a detergent-like complex produced by type II pneumocytes to reduce alveolar surface tension and increase compliance. Surfactant is produced relatively late in foetal life (around 34 weeks' gestation), and so premature babies can develop respiratory distress syndrome. Maternal corticosteroids stimulate surfactant production and thus improve outcome in premature babies.

7 b

Thelarche is the development of breast tissue, which is the first sign of puberty in girls and occurs at an average age of 10.5 years.

8 b

Hyponatraemia and hyperkalaemia occur in Addison's disease. Aldosterone is a mineralocorticoid secreted from the zona glomerulosa of the adrenal cortex. Aldosterone acts to retain water and sodium, and thus low levels of aldosterone in adrenal failure promote hyponatraemia.

9 b

Luteinising hormone (LH) in the male acts on the testes to stimulate Leydig cells to produce testosterone, which is vital in both the development of secondary sexual characteristics and spermatogenesis.

10 a

Pre-proopiomelanocortin (pre-POMC) is a precursor of ACTH, which forms part of the hypothalamic–pituitary axis controlling the production of cortisol.

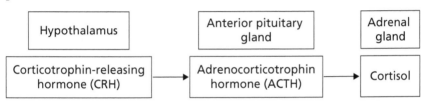

Primary adrenal failure, or Addison's disease, results in high levels of ACTH. This is because high cortisol levels usually feed back negatively on the pituitary to reduce ACTH. Another hormone cleaved from pre-POMC is melanocyte-stimulating hormone. Excess ACTH, as in Addison's, results in melanocyte stimulation and thus hyperpigmentation.

11 e

Prolactin is unique among the pituitary hormones in that it is tonically inhibited by dopamine. Dopamine antagonists, e.g. typical antipsychotic drugs, result in high prolactin levels and can induce galactorrhoea.

12 b

β-hCG levels can be detected in the urine to confirm pregnancy. Excessively high β-hCG may be suggestive of multiple or molar pregnancy.

13 e

Home ovulation-predictor kits work by detecting LH in the urine. The LH surge precedes ovulation by approximately 24 hours, and so this method can be used to predict ovulation and the point of highest fertility.

14 e

Unopposed oestrogens increase the risk of endometrial hyperplasia and malignancy. Progesterone must be given alongside oestrogen therapy in all women with an intact uterus. The risk of endometrial cancer is higher in nulliparous women and those with early menarche and late menopause (increased number of cycles and ovulation).

15 c

The risk of osteoporosis is greatly increased in post-menopausal women as oestrogen levels fall. Hormone-replacement therapy reduces the incidence of osteoporosis, but is not used primarily for this reason. A bisphosphonate is recommended for the prevention of osteoporosis in post-menopausal women.

16 b

The period of the menstrual cycle between the first day of menstruation and ovulation is known as the follicular or proliferative phase, while the 14 days following ovulation is the secretory phase. These terms depict the state of the endometrium in response to the hormonal changes of the cycle. Duration of the proliferative phase is variable depending on cycle length, while the secretory phase remains relatively constant at around 14 days.

17 a

Paracrine is a term used to describe the action by which a hormone acts on local cells via transport in the extracellular fluid, while auto-crine describes the action of a hormone acting on the same cell that produces it.

18 c

Growth hormone is secreted in a pulsatile fashion by the anterior pitu-itary in response to growth hormone–releasing hormone (GHRH). Growth hormone acts via insulin-like growth factors and stimulates growth and well-being. Deficiency of GH in children leads to dwarf-ism, while excess causes gigantism. A pituitary tumour can result in GH overproduction and acromegaly, characterised by classical changes in appearance, large hands and feet, deepening of the voice and weight gain.

19 c

The thyroid axis works to control metabolism. Hypothalamic thyrotrophin-releasing hormone (TRH) stimulates the anterior pitui-tary gland to secrete thyroid stimulating hormone (TSH). Under the influence of TSH, the thyroid gland produces the two thyroid hor-mones, thyroxine (T_4) and triiodothyronine (T_3).

20 a

Prolactin is secreted from the anterior pituitary gland. The most com-mon cause of hyperprolactinaemia is a prolactin-secreting pituitary adenoma (prolactinoma). Excess prolactin can result in galactorrhoea. Local compression of the optic chiasm by the enlarged pituitary can also result in visual field defects, commonly a bitemporal hemianopia (tunnel vision).

21 c

The parafollicular cells of the thyroid produce calcitonin, which plays a role in calcium homeostasis by its effects on bone turnover, intestinal calcium absorption and renal tubule reabsorption. With the opposite effect of parathyroid hormone (PTH), calcitonin acts to decrease blood calcium.

22 d

Calcium metabolism is controlled by vitamin D, parathyroid hormone and calcitonin. Parathyroid hormone (PTH) is secreted by chief cells in the parathyroid gland in response to hypocalcaemia. PTH increases renal tubular and intestinal calcium absorption, as well as promoting osteoclastic reabsorption of calcium from bone.

23 b

Production of the active form of vitamin D, $1,25\text{-}(OH)_2D_3$, occurs via the following pathway.

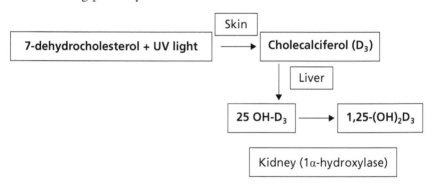

Vitamin D_3 (cholecalciferol) is formed by the photoactivation of 7-dehydrocholesterol in the skin by ultraviolet light. This is then hydroxylated in the liver to form 25 OH-D_3. Finally, the active $1,25\text{-}(OH)_2D_3$ is formed in the kidney by 1α-hydroxylase.

24 a

The pancreas serves as both an endocrine and exocrine organ. Glucagon, insulin and somatostatin are secreted by the pancreas from α-, β- and γ-cells, respectively.

25 b

The hypothalamus–pituitary–thyroid axis is shown below. Each step feeds back negatively on the previous in order to control production.

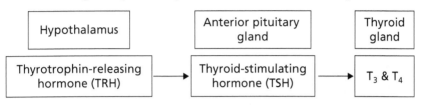

26 b

The adrenal gland is anatomically divided into the cortex and medulla. The outer cortex produces cortisol, aldosterone and androgens, while the medulla secretes catecholamines, noradrenaline and adrenaline. The adrenal cortex is divided into three regions as below.

Cortical layer	Hormone secreted
Zona reticularis	Androgens (e.g. adrenosterone)
Zona fasciculata	Glucocorticoids (e.g. cortisol)
Zona glomerulosa	Mineralocorticoids (e.g. aldosterone)

Theme: The hypothalamic–pituitary axis

1 b

2 d

3 b

4 b

5 e

1 b

The posterior pituitary gland releases both antidiuretic hormone (ADH) and oxytocin. The remainder of the pituitary hormones come from the anterior portion.

Anterior pituitary hormones	Posterior pituitary hormones
Follicle-stimulating hormone	Oxytocin
Luteinising hormone	Antidiuretic hormone (ADH)
Prolactin	
Thyroid-stimulating hormone	
Adrenocorticotrophin-releasing hormone	

2 d

Unlike the other pituitary hormones, prolactin is tonically inhibited by dopamine. Disruption of this inhibition can lead to excess secretion.

3 b

Syndrome of inappropriate ADH secretion (SIADH) can occur secondary to various malignancies, including small-cell lung carcinoma. Biochemically, it results in hyponatraemia, and patients may present with drowsiness, irritability or even coma.

4 b

Diabetes insipidus (DI) is a disorder characterised by the inability to secrete or utilise ADH. This results in the inability to concentrate the urine and the production of large volumes of dilute urine and dehydration. DI may be cranial (inability to secrete ADH) or nephro-genic (inability of ADH to act on the nephron).

5 e
Gonadotrophin-releasing hormone (GnRH) controls the secretion of FSH and LH from the anterior pituitary gland. They are essential in the control of the menstrual cycle and fertility in women and testo-sterone production and spermatogenesis in men.

Theme: The menstrual cycle

1 k

2 j

3 i

4 e

5 d

1 k

Endometrial tissue of the uterus is hormone-sensitive in order to prepare for implantation or menstruation. 'Unopposed oestrogens' (i.e. oestrogen therapy without progesterone) can lead to endometrial hyperplasia and malignancy.

2 j

An average menstrual cycle lasts for 28 days, with day 1 being the first day of menstruation and day 14 the time of ovulation.

3 i

Day 21 progesterone level can be measured to detect ovulation in 28-day cycles. As the luteal phase of the cycle remains constant, the mid-luteal level will always be 7 days before the end of the cycle (i.e. 8 days before the start of menstruation).

4 e

GnRH is secreted by the hypothalamus to control the secretion of the anterior pituitary hormones, follicle-stimulating hormone (FSH) and luteinising hormone (LH).

5 d

Progesterone optimises the uterus for pregnancy. The corpus luteum formed from the post-ovulatory follicle produces progesterone before the placenta takes over at about week 10.

Theme: Water and electrolyte balance

1 c

2 h

3 a

4 g

5 h

1 c

Osmolarity is the major factor controlling the release of antidiuretic hormone (ADH). An increase in osmolarity is sensed by hypothalamic osmoreceptors. ADH results in the insertion of aquaporin channels to promote water conservation at the collecting duct and thus reduces osmolarity. A reduction in plasma volume can also lead to ADH secretion, but a greater change is needed (approximately 15% reduction).

2 h

Aldosterone promotes retention of sodium and water. By antagonising this effect, spironolactone creates a diuresis, hence its therapeutic use in congestive cardiac failure.

3 a

Antidiuretic hormone (ADH) is released from the posterior pituitary gland in order to conserve water and sodium, by increasing the permeability of the collecting duct to water, thus allowing more reabsorption. Its actions include augmenting the release of aldosterone, which promotes the retention of salt and water.

4 g

Furosemide acts on the loop of Henle and is therefore known as a loop diuretic. It works by blocking the $Na^+/K^+/2Cl^-$ cotransporter at the thick ascending limb to inhibit active Na^+ absorption.

5 h

Spironolactone is an aldosterone antagonist and a potassium-sparing diuretic. Care must be taken when prescribing diuretics. If given alongside an ACE inhibitor, spironolactone can result in dangerous hyperkalaemia.

Theme: Diabetes mellitus

1 d

2 e

3 f

4 i

5 h

1 d

Diabetic ketoacidosis (DKA) is a potentially life-threatening complication of type I diabetes resulting from insulin deficiency. A state of uncontrolled catabolism results in high levels of circulating blood glucose, osmotic diuresis and dehydration. Peripheral lipolysis leads to an increase in free fatty acids. Hepatic conversion of fatty acids to acidic ketones leads to a state of metabolic acidosis.

2 e

Type I diabetes mellitus results from autoimmune destruction of the β-islet cells, resulting in impaired insulin secretion. It usually presents in childhood with the characteristic triad of weight loss, polyuria and polydipsia.

3 f

Type II diabetes mellitus has a later onset than type I and is associated with obesity resulting from peripheral insulin resistance. In the later stages, amyloid formation and islet destruction can occur, necessitating insulin therapy.

4 i

Glucagon is secreted by α-islets cells of the pancreas. It stimulates gluconeogenesis and mobilises hepatic glycogen stores to increase blood glucose levels.

5 h

Insulin is secreted by β-cells to lower elevated blood glucose by facilitating uptake by fat and muscle. Diabetes mellitus results from impaired insulin production or action resulting in chronically high blood glucose.

Section 5: Fluid regulation and the kidneys

1 e

The kidneys have a wide range of functions which extend far beyond excretion of waste substances. Their role in acid–base and fluid balance, osmolarity and erythropoiesis will all be tested in the questions in this section.

2 a

The renal tubule follows Ussing's model of epithelial transport. In absorptive cells following Ussing's model, the primary driving event is the Na^+/K^+ ATPase pump on the basolateral membrane of the cell. This acts to keep intracellular Na^+ concentration low, thereby allowing Na^+ to enter the cell down its concentration gradient across the apical membrane. This facilitates the reabsorption of sodium (and therefore water), as Na^+ crosses the apical membrane and the basolateral membrane, namely 'transepithelial' transport.

3 e

Antidiuretic hormone, as the name indicates, acts in the opposite way to diuretics, thereby retaining water. It facilitates this by action at vasopressin (V_2) receptors, leading to the insertion of aquaporin II channels in the collecting duct. They increase water permeability of the collecting duct, and therefore facilitate water conservation.

4 e

Osmoreceptors in the hypothalamus detect changes in plasma osmolarity. An increase of just 1% is sufficient to trigger secretion of ADH, which increases water reabsorption and thus decreases osmolarity.

5 b

Erythropoietin is secreted in response to hypoxia in order to increase red cell production. This acts to increase blood oxygen-carrying capacity in hypoxic conditions, e.g. at altitude when atmospheric partial pressure of O_2 is lower.

6 e

Furosemide is a loop diuretic commonly used in the management of hypertension. It is also effective in treating peripheral and pulmonary oedema, secondary to heart failure. Loop diuretics act by inhibiting chloride reabsorption in the ascending limb of the loop of Henle. This leads to natriuresis, and because water follows sodium, diuresis.

7 b

Loop diuretics promote diuresis by acting at the $Na^+/K^+/2Cl^-$ cotransporter. Inhibition of the $Na^+/K^+/2Cl^-$ results in potassium excretion, which can lead to hypokalaemia if potassium supplements are not given.

8 c

The renin–angiotensin–aldosterone (RAA) axis plays a vital role in the regulation of blood pressure and fluid balance. Angiotensinogen is converted to angiotensin I by renin, which is secreted by the juxtaglomerular apparatus of the kidney in response to reduced perfusion.

9 e

Aldosterone is secreted in response to increased angiotensin II and results in reabsorption of sodium and water, thus increasing blood volume and raising blood pressure. Many antihypertensives act on this system and reduce blood pressure by inhibiting the RAA axis at various stages.

10 e

Body fluid pH must be maintained within a very narrow range in order to optimise enzyme function. A small deviation from the normal range can prove life-threatening. The kidneys play a vital role in the maintenance of acid–base balance. Renal compensation to an acid–base disorder usually takes 2–3 days (respiratory compensation is more immediate). The kidneys minimize pH disturbance in acidosis by increasing acid excretion and HCO_3^- reabsorption. In normal conditions, over 99% of the filtered HCO_3^- is reabsorbed, mainly in the proximal tubules. In the proximal tubule, H^+ secretion occurs via the Na^+/H^+ counter transporter. In the late distal and collecting tubules, H^+ ions are secreted by active transport, i.e. H^+-ATPase. H^+ secretion can be augmented to increase tubular H^+ concentration by as much as 900-fold.

11 a

Under normal circumstances, glomerular filtrate is principally identical to plasma without the proteins, which are too large to pass through the filtration barrier. This barrier is made up of three components: interdigitating pedicels from podocyte cells, a negatively charged basement membrane and the fenestrated endothelial capillary cells.

12 d

The bladder is distensible and can store urine by expanding and contracting. At around 250 mL, most adults get the sensation of having a full bladder, although it can store in excess of 500 mL. The detrusor muscle contracts and internal sphincter relaxes via involuntary autonomic control when the bladder is ready to empty. In a healthy adult, micturition is a voluntary action via relaxation of the external sphincter.

13 b

An average, healthy man passes an average of 0.5 mL/kg/hour. Therefore, a 70-kg man would be expected to pass 0.5 × 70 = 35 mL every hour. Low volumes of urine (oliguria) suggest acute renal failure, and the cause must be found to prevent irreversible kidney damage.

14 b

The detrusor muscle is made up of smooth muscle which relaxes to fill. It is lined with transitional epithelium. The bladder lies extraperitoneally, but as it expands it enters the abdominal cavity.

15 c

Approximately 20% of cardiac output supplies the kidneys. Urine output is a very useful sign of circulatory compromise and should be monitored carefully in the acutely unwell patient.

16 c

Glomerular filtration takes place between the glomerulus and Bowman's capsule. The filter prevents the passage of proteins from the blood into the filtrate by the presence of pores (too small for the large protein molecules) and negative charge on the basement membrane, which repel the molecules.

17 e

In order to measure glomerular filtration rate (GFR) by the clearance of solution X, it must be that the volume of solution X is not affected by the kidney itself. For example, if the nephron either secreted or absorbed solution X, the amount cleared would not reflect the filtration rate. Inulin obeys all of the above rules and thus can be used to measure GFR.

18 c

Angiotensin-converting enzyme (ACE) coverts angiotensin I to II and plays a role in the renin–angiotensin–aldosterone axis and fluid balance. ACE is synthesised in the lungs.

19 d

Aldosterone is produced by the zona glomerulosa of the adrenal cortex and acts on the renal tubules to retain sodium and water. Its production is stimulated by the presence of angiotensin II.

20 c

Starling forces drive glomerular filtration. Forces promoting filtration include capillary hydrostatic pressure and oncotic pressure in the Bowman's capsule. Both promote the movement of filtrate from the capillary lumen to the capsular space.

21 a

Oncotic pressure is driven by the presence of protein in the capillary lumen. The oncotic pressure in the capillary lumen is higher than that in the Bowman's capsule, thus capillary oncotic pressure promotes movement from the capsular space to the capillary; it opposes filtration.

22 a

In situations of dehydration, the nephron will aim to conserve water by the actions of the renin–angiotensin–aldosterone axis. Antidiuretic hormone will be stimulated to increase collecting-duct water permeability, leading to the production of small amounts of concentrated urine.

23 d

Diabetes insipidus (DI) is a condition in which there is underproduction (cranial DI) or failure of action (nephrogenic DI) of antidiuretic hormone. This prevents the nephron from being able to conserve water, and leads to the frequent production of large volumes of dilute urine.

24 d

In order to maintain a relatively constant GFR, the nephron has a mechanism of autoregulation, whereby an increase in blood pressure is detected by increased stretch in the wall of the afferent arteriole, leading to smooth muscle contraction of the arteriole, thus preventing a rise in GFR with the increase in blood pressure.

25 c

Approximately one fifth of the filtrate formed by glomerular filtration is reabsorbed at the loop of Henle.

26 e

Renal failure can be divided into three causes: prerenal, renal or intrinsic, and postrenal. Options a and b are both causes of prerenal failure; there is reduced renal perfusion. Options c and d are causes of intrinsic renal damage. Obstruction of the renal tract makes up the postrenal cause, and can be due to renal calculi, pelvic tumours or prostatic enlargement.

Theme: Acid–base balance and the kidneys

1 a

2 d

3 e

4 h

5 j

1 a

An acidosis can be compensated by respiratory and renal means. A metabolic acidosis can be compensated by increasing the rate of breathing. Hyperventilating allows carbon dioxide to be blown off, increasing the $HCO_3^- : CO_2$ ratio, which according to the Henderson–Hasselbach equation, increases the pH:

$$pH = pKa + \log \frac{(HCO_3^-)}{CO_2}$$

pKa = the acid dissociation constant

2 d

Metabolic alkalosis results in an increase in pH due to increased plasma bicarbonate or chloride, or decreased hydrogen or potassium ions. Common causes of metabolic alkalosis in hospital include vomiting, the use of diuretics (e.g. furosemide) and nasogastric suction. Vomiting and bulimia result in gastric acid loss and resultant metabolic alkalosis.

3 e

Respiratory acidosis results in an increase in pH due to carbon dioxide retention. This may be secondary to hypoventilation, or poor gaseous exchange at the alveoli. Opiate overdose results in respiratory depression. Naloxone can be given to reverse the effects of opiate toxicity.

4   h

The anion gap is extremely useful in assessing the cause of a metabolic acidosis and can be calculated using the following formula:

$$\text{Anion gap} = (Na^+ + K^+) - (HCO_3^- + Cl^-)$$

Because there are more positive ions (anions) than negative ions (cations), the normal range of the anion gap is 10–18 mmol/L. If the anion gap is increased, it can be deduced that the metabolic acidosis is due to the presence of unmeasured anions. Causes of a metabolic acidosis with a high anion gap include lactic acidosis, diabetic ketoacidosis and aspirin overdose.

5   j

Causes of metabolic acidosis with a normal anion gap include renal tubular acidosis and diarrhoea. Renal tubular acidosis (RTA) results in a decrease in plasma pH and may be secondary to structural, immunological or drug-induced tubular damage.

Theme: The renin–angiotensin–aldosterone axis

1 a

2 f

3 d

4 j

5 h

1 a

A reduction in circulating volume results in renin release from granular cells of the kidney. Renin converts angiotensinogen into angiotensin I. Angiotensin-converting enzyme (ACE) catalyses the conversion of angiotensin I to angiotensin II. Angiotensin II promotes an increase in extracellular volume and blood pressure by vasoconstriction and stimulates the release of adrenal aldosterone, which promotes salt and water retention.

2 f

Angiotensin II is formed when extracellular volume is depleted and causes vasoconstriction, via the actions of renin and angiotensin-converting enzyme. Angiotensin II promotes increased circulating volume and blood pressure by stimulating the thirst centres, ADH and aldosterone release. All these factors promote the retention of salt and water and reduce excretion.

3 d

Atrial natriuretic peptide (ANP) acts to inhibit reabsorption and increase excretion, thus the opposite effect of the renin–angiotensin–aldosterone system. It does this by inhibiting the effects of angiotensin II on tubular transport and inhibits both renin and aldosterone release.

4 j

Baroreceptors in the carotid sinus and aortic arch detect a reduction in extracellular volume and signal to the medulla. Reduced circulating volume stimulates sodium reabsorption, the release of renin and vasoconstriction. Large falls in extracellular volume (over 15%) also trigger release of ADH from the posterior pituitary gland, which causes the collecting duct to become more permeable to water.

5 h

A change in plasma osmolality as small as 1% triggers ADH release from the posterior pituitary gland. ADH stimulates the insertion of aquaporin II channels in the collecting duct, increasing its permeability to water.

Theme: Renal transplantation

1 m

2 b

3 f

4 h

5 l

1 m

In order to prevent graft rejection, the recipient undergoes immunosuppressive therapy. The resulting high infection risk is one of the major complications of transplant surgery. Co-trimoxazole and antibiotic prophylaxis are given to prevent *Pneumocystis carinii* pneumonia (PCP) and other infections.

2 b

Arteriovenous fistulae are constructed by a vascular surgeon to allow haemodialysis to take place. The radial or brachial arteries are used and attached to a vein. At least 6 weeks must be given for the AV fistula to develop so that the vein 'arterialises'. Complications of haemodialysis include hypotension, infection and thrombosis.

3 f

The commonest cause of chronic renal failure in the UK is diabetic nephropathy. Sedentary lifestyle and poor diet increase the risk of obesity and diabetes. Tight control of blood glucose and blood pressure help to prevent the development of nephropathy.

4 h

A regimen of corticosteroids and immunosuppressants are given to reduce the risk of graft rejection. Infections such as tuberculosis and PCP can occur, and the risk of septicaemia is high. Live vaccines should be avoided and prophylactic antibiotics given.

5 1

The transplanted kidney can be palpated in the iliac fossa, and the scar is known as the 'hockey stick' scar, due to its characteristic shape.

Theme: Monitoring and maintaining fluid balance

1 k

2 i

3 a

4 f

5 e

1 k

Osmoreceptors in the hypothalamus detect changes in osmolarity by either shrinking or swelling with osmosis. An increase in osmolarity is sensed and signalled to the posterior pituitary gland, where ADH is secreted from the neurohypophyses or posterior pituitary gland, in order to increase water permeability of the collecting duct to dilute and reduce plasma osmolarity.

2 i

ADH is secreted from the posterior pituitary gland in response to increased osmolarity as detected in the hypothalamus. The only other hormone secreted from the posterior part of the pituitary is oxytocin, while follicle-stimulating hormone, luteinising hormone, growth hormone, thyroid-stimulating hormone, adrenocorticotrophin hormone and prolactin are all products of the anterior pituitary gland.

3 a

Autoregulation is the process by which the kidney self-maintains glomerular filtration rate (GFR) irrespective of changes in arterial pressure. It occurs via myogenic mechanisms, in which the increased stretch of arterioles due to increased hydrostatic pressure causes smooth muscle contraction. Additionally, the macula densa senses the increase in GFR because the distal flow rate also increases. This method stimulates constriction of the afferent arteriole, which prevents GFR from rising with the rise in blood pressure.

4 f

Granular cells in the juxtaglomerular apparatus (JGA) are responsible for the secretion of renin in response to a low circulating volume. Renin stimulates the renin–angiotensin–aldosterone axis, which ultimately results in water and sodium retention and an increase in systemic vascular resistance.

5 e

Cardiac output is dependent on heart rate and stroke volume (i.e. cardiac output is equivalent to stroke volume multiplied by heart rate). A reduction in cardiac output leads to reduced renal perfusion, resulting in the common problem of coexisting renal and cardiac disease, when fluid balance becomes very tricky!

Index